Hydroxycitric Acid

A MEDICAL DICTIONARY, BIBLIOGRAPHY,
AND ANNOTATED RESEARCH GUIDE TO
INTERNET REFERENCES

JAMES N. PARKER, M.D.
AND PHILIP M. PARKER, PH.D., EDITORS

ICON Health Publications
ICON Group International, Inc.
4370 La Jolla Village Drive, 4th Floor
San Diego, CA 92122 USA

Copyright ©2004 by ICON Group International, Inc.

Copyright ©2004 by ICON Group International, Inc. All rights reserved. This book is protected by copyright. No part of it may be reproduced, stored in a retrieval system, or transmitted in any form or by any means, electronic, mechanical, photocopying, recording, or otherwise, without written permission from the publisher.

Printed in the United States of America.

Last digit indicates print number: 10 9 8 7 6 4 5 3 2 1

Publisher, Health Care: Philip Parker, Ph.D.
Editor(s): James Parker, M.D., Philip Parker, Ph.D.

Publisher's note: The ideas, procedures, and suggestions contained in this book are not intended for the diagnosis or treatment of a health problem. As new medical or scientific information becomes available from academic and clinical research, recommended treatments and drug therapies may undergo changes. The authors, editors, and publisher have attempted to make the information in this book up to date and accurate in accord with accepted standards at the time of publication. The authors, editors, and publisher are not responsible for errors or omissions or for consequences from application of the book, and make no warranty, expressed or implied, in regard to the contents of this book. Any practice described in this book should be applied by the reader in accordance with professional standards of care used in regard to the unique circumstances that may apply in each situation. The reader is advised to always check product information (package inserts) for changes and new information regarding dosage and contraindications before prescribing any drug or pharmacological product. Caution is especially urged when using new or infrequently ordered drugs, herbal remedies, vitamins and supplements, alternative therapies, complementary therapies and medicines, and integrative medical treatments.

Cataloging-in-Publication Data

Parker, James N., 1961-
Parker, Philip M., 1960-

Hydroxycitric Acid: A Medical Dictionary, Bibliography, and Annotated Research Guide to Internet References / James N. Parker and Philip M. Parker, editors
        p.   cm.
Includes bibliographical references, glossary, and index.
ISBN: 0-497-00562-X
1. Hydroxycitric Acid-Popular works. I. Title.

Disclaimer

This publication is not intended to be used for the diagnosis or treatment of a health problem. It is sold with the understanding that the publisher, editors, and authors are not engaging in the rendering of medical, psychological, financial, legal, or other professional services.

References to any entity, product, service, or source of information that may be contained in this publication should not be considered an endorsement, either direct or implied, by the publisher, editors, or authors. ICON Group International, Inc., the editors, and the authors are not responsible for the content of any Web pages or publications referenced in this publication.

Copyright Notice

If a physician wishes to copy limited passages from this book for patient use, this right is automatically granted without written permission from ICON Group International, Inc. (ICON Group). However, all of ICON Group publications have copyrights. With exception to the above, copying our publications in whole or in part, for whatever reason, is a violation of copyright laws and can lead to penalties and fines. Should you want to copy tables, graphs, or other materials, please contact us to request permission (E-mail: iconedit@san.rr.com). ICON Group often grants permission for very limited reproduction of our publications for internal use, press releases, and academic research. Such reproduction requires confirmed permission from ICON Group International, Inc. **The disclaimer above must accompany all reproductions, in whole or in part, of this book.**

Acknowledgements

The collective knowledge generated from academic and applied research summarized in various references has been critical in the creation of this book which is best viewed as a comprehensive compilation and collection of information prepared by various official agencies which produce publications on hydroxycitric acid. Books in this series draw from various agencies and institutions associated with the United States Department of Health and Human Services, and in particular, the Office of the Secretary of Health and Human Services (OS), the Administration for Children and Families (ACF), the Administration on Aging (AOA), the Agency for Healthcare Research and Quality (AHRQ), the Agency for Toxic Substances and Disease Registry (ATSDR), the Centers for Disease Control and Prevention (CDC), the Food and Drug Administration (FDA), the Healthcare Financing Administration (HCFA), the Health Resources and Services Administration (HRSA), the Indian Health Service (IHS), the institutions of the National Institutes of Health (NIH), the Program Support Center (PSC), and the Substance Abuse and Mental Health Services Administration (SAMHSA). In addition to these sources, information gathered from the National Library of Medicine, the United States Patent Office, the European Union, and their related organizations has been invaluable in the creation of this book. Some of the work represented was financially supported by the Research and Development Committee at INSEAD. This support is gratefully acknowledged. Finally, special thanks are owed to Tiffany Freeman for her excellent editorial support.

About the Editors

James N. Parker, M.D.

Dr. James N. Parker received his Bachelor of Science degree in Psychobiology from the University of California, Riverside and his M.D. from the University of California, San Diego. In addition to authoring numerous research publications, he has lectured at various academic institutions. Dr. Parker is the medical editor for health books by ICON Health Publications.

Philip M. Parker, Ph.D.

Philip M. Parker is the Eli Lilly Chair Professor of Innovation, Business and Society at INSEAD (Fontainebleau, France and Singapore). Dr. Parker has also been Professor at the University of California, San Diego and has taught courses at Harvard University, the Hong Kong University of Science and Technology, the Massachusetts Institute of Technology, Stanford University, and UCLA. Dr. Parker is the associate editor for ICON Health Publications.

About ICON Health Publications

To discover more about ICON Health Publications, simply check with your preferred online booksellers, including Barnes&Noble.com and Amazon.com which currently carry all of our titles. Or, feel free to contact us directly for bulk purchases or institutional discounts:

ICON Group International, Inc.
4370 La Jolla Village Drive, Fourth Floor
San Diego, CA 92122 USA
Fax: 858-546-4341
Web site: **www.icongrouponline.com/health**

Table of Contents

FORWARD	1
CHAPTER 1. STUDIES ON HYDROXYCITRIC ACID	3
Overview	3
Federally Funded Research on Hydroxycitric Acid	3
The National Library of Medicine: PubMed	3
CHAPTER 2. NUTRITION AND HYDROXYCITRIC ACID	5
Overview	5
Finding Nutrition Studies on Hydroxycitric Acid	5
Federal Resources on Nutrition	6
Additional Web Resources	7
CHAPTER 3. ALTERNATIVE MEDICINE AND HYDROXYCITRIC ACID	9
Overview	9
National Center for Complementary and Alternative Medicine	9
Additional Web Resources	12
General References	13
CHAPTER 4. PATENTS ON HYDROXYCITRIC ACID	15
Overview	15
Patents on Hydroxycitric Acid	15
Patent Applications on Hydroxycitric Acid	19
Keeping Current	21
APPENDIX A. PHYSICIAN RESOURCES	25
Overview	25
NIH Guidelines	25
NIH Databases	27
Other Commercial Databases	29
APPENDIX B. PATIENT RESOURCES	31
Overview	31
Patient Guideline Sources	31
Finding Associations	32
APPENDIX C. FINDING MEDICAL LIBRARIES	35
Overview	35
Preparation	35
Finding a Local Medical Library	35
Medical Libraries in the U.S. and Canada	35
ONLINE GLOSSARIES	**41**
Online Dictionary Directories	41
HYDROXYCITRIC ACID DICTIONARY	**43**
INDEX	**55**

FORWARD

In March 2001, the National Institutes of Health issued the following warning: "The number of Web sites offering health-related resources grows every day. Many sites provide valuable information, while others may have information that is unreliable or misleading."[1] Furthermore, because of the rapid increase in Internet-based information, many hours can be wasted searching, selecting, and printing. Since only the smallest fraction of information dealing with hydroxycitric acid is indexed in search engines, such as **www.google.com** or others, a non-systematic approach to Internet research can be not only time consuming, but also incomplete. This book was created for medical professionals, students, and members of the general public who want to know as much as possible about hydroxycitric acid, using the most advanced research tools available and spending the least amount of time doing so.

In addition to offering a structured and comprehensive bibliography, the pages that follow will tell you where and how to find reliable information covering virtually all topics related to hydroxycitric acid, from the essentials to the most advanced areas of research. Public, academic, government, and peer-reviewed research studies are emphasized. Various abstracts are reproduced to give you some of the latest official information available to date on hydroxycitric acid. Abundant guidance is given on how to obtain free-of-charge primary research results via the Internet. **While this book focuses on the field of medicine, when some sources provide access to non-medical information relating to hydroxycitric acid, these are noted in the text.**

E-book and electronic versions of this book are fully interactive with each of the Internet sites mentioned (clicking on a hyperlink automatically opens your browser to the site indicated). If you are using the hard copy version of this book, you can access a cited Web site by typing the provided Web address directly into your Internet browser. You may find it useful to refer to synonyms or related terms when accessing these Internet databases. **NOTE:** At the time of publication, the Web addresses were functional. However, some links may fail due to URL address changes, which is a common occurrence on the Internet.

For readers unfamiliar with the Internet, detailed instructions are offered on how to access electronic resources. For readers unfamiliar with medical terminology, a comprehensive glossary is provided. For readers without access to Internet resources, a directory of medical libraries, that have or can locate references cited here, is given. We hope these resources will prove useful to the widest possible audience seeking information on hydroxycitric acid.

The Editors

---

[1] From the NIH, National Cancer Institute (NCI): **http://www.cancer.gov/cancerinfo/ten-things-to-know**.

CHAPTER 1. STUDIES ON HYDROXYCITRIC ACID

Overview

In this chapter, we will show you how to locate peer-reviewed references and studies on hydroxycitric acid.

Federally Funded Research on Hydroxycitric Acid

The U.S. Government supports a variety of research studies relating to hydroxycitric acid. These studies are tracked by the Office of Extramural Research at the National Institutes of Health.[2] CRISP (Computerized Retrieval of Information on Scientific Projects) is a searchable database of federally funded biomedical research projects conducted at universities, hospitals, and other institutions.

Search the CRISP Web site at http://crisp.cit.nih.gov/crisp/crisp_query.generate_screen. You will have the option to perform targeted searches by various criteria, including geography, date, and topics related to hydroxycitric acid.

For most of the studies, the agencies reporting into CRISP provide summaries or abstracts. As opposed to clinical trial research using patients, many federally funded studies use animals or simulated models to explore hydroxycitric acid.

The National Library of Medicine: PubMed

One of the quickest and most comprehensive ways to find academic studies in both English and other languages is to use PubMed, maintained by the National Library of Medicine.[3]

---

[2] Healthcare projects are funded by the National Institutes of Health (NIH), Substance Abuse and Mental Health Services (SAMHSA), Health Resources and Services Administration (HRSA), Food and Drug Administration (FDA), Centers for Disease Control and Prevention (CDCP), Agency for Healthcare Research and Quality (AHRQ), and Office of Assistant Secretary of Health (OASH).

[3] PubMed was developed by the National Center for Biotechnology Information (NCBI) at the National Library of Medicine (NLM) at the National Institutes of Health (NIH). The PubMed database was developed in conjunction with publishers of biomedical literature as a search tool for accessing literature citations and linking to full-text

The advantage of PubMed over previously mentioned sources is that it covers a greater number of domestic and foreign references. It is also free to use. If the publisher has a Web site that offers full text of its journals, PubMed will provide links to that site, as well as to sites offering other related data. User registration, a subscription fee, or some other type of fee may be required to access the full text of articles in some journals.

To generate your own bibliography of studies dealing with hydroxycitric acid, simply go to the PubMed Web site at **http://www.ncbi.nlm.nih.gov/pubmed**. Type "hydroxycitric acid" (or synonyms) into the search box, and click "Go." The following is the type of output you can expect from PubMed for hydroxycitric acid (hyperlinks lead to article summaries):

- **(-)-Hydroxycitric acid ingestion increases fat utilization during exercise in untrained women.**
  Author(s): Lim K, Ryu S, Nho HS, Choi SK, Kwon T, Suh H, So J, Tomita K, Okuhara Y, Shigematsu N.
  Source: J Nutr Sci Vitaminol (Tokyo). 2003 June; 49(3): 163-7.
  http://www.ncbi.nlm.nih.gov/entrez/query.fcgi?cmd=Retrieve&db=pubmed&dopt=Abstract&list_uids=12953793

- **Chemistry and biochemistry of (-)-hydroxycitric acid from Garcinia.**
  Author(s): Jena BS, Jayaprakasha GK, Singh RP, Sakariah KK.
  Source: Journal of Agricultural and Food Chemistry. 2002 January 2; 50(1): 10-22. Review.
  http://www.ncbi.nlm.nih.gov/entrez/query.fcgi?cmd=Retrieve&db=pubmed&dopt=Abstract&list_uids=11754536

- **Effects of (-)-hydroxycitric acid on appetitive variables.**
  Author(s): Mattes RD, Bormann L.
  Source: Physiology & Behavior. 2000 October 1-15; 71(1-2): 87-94.
  http://www.ncbi.nlm.nih.gov/entrez/query.fcgi?cmd=Retrieve&db=pubmed&dopt=Abstract&list_uids=11134690

- **Safety assessment of (-)-hydroxycitric acid and Super CitriMax, a novel calcium/potassium salt.**
  Author(s): Soni MG, Burdock GA, Preuss HG, Stohs SJ, Ohia SE, Bagchi D.
  Source: Food and Chemical Toxicology : an International Journal Published for the British Industrial Biological Research Association. 2004 September; 42(9): 1513-29. Review.
  http://www.ncbi.nlm.nih.gov/entrez/query.fcgi?cmd=Retrieve&db=pubmed&dopt=Abstract&list_uids=15234082

---

journal articles at Web sites of participating publishers. Publishers that participate in PubMed supply NLM with their citations electronically prior to or at the time of publication.

CHAPTER 2. NUTRITION AND HYDROXYCITRIC ACID

Overview

In this chapter, we will show you how to find studies dedicated specifically to nutrition and hydroxycitric acid.

Finding Nutrition Studies on Hydroxycitric Acid

The National Institutes of Health's Office of Dietary Supplements (ODS) offers a searchable bibliographic database called the IBIDS (International Bibliographic Information on Dietary Supplements; National Institutes of Health, Building 31, Room 1B29, 31 Center Drive, MSC 2086, Bethesda, Maryland 20892-2086, Tel: 301-435-2920, Fax: 301-480-1845, E-mail: ods@nih.gov). The IBIDS contains over 460,000 scientific citations and summaries about dietary supplements and nutrition as well as references to published international, scientific literature on dietary supplements such as vitamins, minerals, and botanicals.[4] The IBIDS includes references and citations to both human and animal research studies.

As a service of the ODS, access to the IBIDS database is available free of charge at the following Web address: **http://ods.od.nih.gov/databases/ibids.html**. After entering the search area, you have three choices: (1) IBIDS Consumer Database, (2) Full IBIDS Database, or (3) Peer Reviewed Citations Only.

Now that you have selected a database, click on the "Advanced" tab. An advanced search allows you to retrieve up to 100 fully explained references in a comprehensive format. Type "hydroxycitric acid" (or synonyms) into the search box, and click "Go." To narrow the search, you can also select the "Title" field.

---

[4] Adapted from **http://ods.od.nih.gov**. IBIDS is produced by the Office of Dietary Supplements (ODS) at the National Institutes of Health to assist the public, healthcare providers, educators, and researchers in locating credible, scientific information on dietary supplements. IBIDS was developed and will be maintained through an interagency partnership with the Food and Nutrition Information Center of the National Agricultural Library, U.S. Department of Agriculture.

The following information is typical of that found when using the "Full IBIDS Database" to search for "hydroxycitric acid" (or a synonym):

- **Determination of (-) hydroxycitric acid in commercial samples of Garcinia cambogia extract by liquid chromatography with ultraviolet detection.**
  Source: Jayaprakasha, G.K. Sakariah, K.K. J-liq-chromatogr-relat-technol. Monticello, NY : Marcel Dekker, Inc. 2000. volume 23 (6) page 915-923. 1082-6076

- **Effect of hydroxycitric acid on serotonin release from isolated rat brain cortex.**
  Author(s): Department of Pharmacy Sciences, School of Pharmacy and Allied Health Professions, Creighton University, Omaha, NE 68178, USA.
  Source: Ohia S, E Awe S, O LeDay A, M Opere C, A Bagchi, D Res-Commun-Mol-Pathol-Pharmacol. 2001 Mar-April; 109(3-4): 210-6 1078-0297

- **Safety and mechanism of appetite suppression by a novel hydroxycitric acid extract (HCA-SX).**
  Author(s): Department of Pharmacy Sciences, Creighton University School of Pharmacy and Allied Health Professions, Omaha, NE 68178, USA. seohia@creighton.edu
  Source: Ohia, S E Opere, C A LeDay, A M Bagchi, M Bagchi, D Stohs, S J Mol-Cell-Biochem. 2002 September; 238(1-2): 89-103 0300-8177

Federal Resources on Nutrition

In addition to the IBIDS, the United States Department of Health and Human Services (HHS) and the United States Department of Agriculture (USDA) provide many sources of information on general nutrition and health. Recommended resources include:

- healthfinder®, HHS's gateway to health information, including diet and nutrition: **http://www.healthfinder.gov/scripts/SearchContext.asp?topic=238&page=0**

- The United States Department of Agriculture's Web site dedicated to nutrition information: **www.nutrition.gov**

- The Food and Drug Administration's Web site for federal food safety information: **www.foodsafety.gov**

- The National Action Plan on Overweight and Obesity sponsored by the United States Surgeon General: **http://www.surgeongeneral.gov/topics/obesity/**

- The Center for Food Safety and Applied Nutrition has an Internet site sponsored by the Food and Drug Administration and the Department of Health and Human Services: **http://vm.cfsan.fda.gov/**

- Center for Nutrition Policy and Promotion sponsored by the United States Department of Agriculture: **http://www.usda.gov/cnpp/**

- Food and Nutrition Information Center, National Agricultural Library sponsored by the United States Department of Agriculture: **http://www.nal.usda.gov/fnic/**

- Food and Nutrition Service sponsored by the United States Department of Agriculture: **http://www.fns.usda.gov/fns/**

Additional Web Resources

A number of additional Web sites offer encyclopedic information covering food and nutrition. The following is a representative sample:

- AOL: http://search.aol.com/cat.adp?id=174&layer=&from=subcats
- Family Village: http://www.familyvillage.wisc.edu/med_nutrition.html
- Google: http://directory.google.com/Top/Health/Nutrition/
- Healthnotes: http://www.healthnotes.com/
- Open Directory Project: http://dmoz.org/Health/Nutrition/
- Yahoo.com: http://dir.yahoo.com/Health/Nutrition/
- WebMD®Health: http://my.webmd.com/nutrition
- WholeHealthMD.com: http://www.wholehealthmd.com/reflib/0,1529,00.html

The following is a specific Web list relating to hydroxycitric acid; please note that any particular subject below may indicate either a therapeutic use, or a contraindication (potential danger), and does not reflect an official recommendation:

- **Food and Diet**

    Weight Management Index
    Source: Healthnotes, Inc.; www.healthnotes.com

CHAPTER 3. ALTERNATIVE MEDICINE AND HYDROXYCITRIC ACID

Overview

In this chapter, we will begin by introducing you to official information sources on complementary and alternative medicine (CAM) relating to hydroxycitric acid. At the conclusion of this chapter, we will provide additional sources.

National Center for Complementary and Alternative Medicine

The National Center for Complementary and Alternative Medicine (NCCAM) of the National Institutes of Health (http://nccam.nih.gov/) has created a link to the National Library of Medicine's databases to facilitate research for articles that specifically relate to hydroxycitric acid and complementary medicine. To search the database, go to the following Web site: **http://www.nlm.nih.gov/nccam/camonpubmed.html**. Select "CAM on PubMed." Enter "hydroxycitric acid" (or synonyms) into the search box. Click "Go." The following references provide information on particular aspects of complementary and alternative medicine that are related to hydroxycitric acid:

- **(-)-Hydroxycitric acid does not affect energy expenditure and substrate oxidation in adult males in a post-absorptive state.**
  Author(s): Kriketos AD, Thompson HR, Greene H, Hill JO.
  Source: International Journal of Obesity and Related Metabolic Disorders : Journal of the International Association for the Study of Obesity. 1999 August; 23(8): 867-73.
  http://www.ncbi.nlm.nih.gov/entrez/query.fcgi?cmd=Retrieve&db=pubmed&dopt=Abstract&list_uids=10490789

- **Alternative therapies: Part I. Depression, diabetes, obesity.**
  Author(s): Morelli V, Zoorob RJ.
  Source: American Family Physician. 2000 September 1; 62(5): 1051-60. Review.
  http://www.ncbi.nlm.nih.gov/entrez/query.fcgi?cmd=Retrieve&db=pubmed&dopt=Abstract&list_uids=10997530

- **Body weight and abdominal fat gene expression profile in response to a novel hydroxycitric acid-based dietary supplement.**
  Author(s): Roy S, Rink C, Khanna S, Phillips C, Bagchi D, Bagchi M, Sen CK.
  Source: Gene Expression. 2004; 11(5-6): 251-62.
  http://www.ncbi.nlm.nih.gov/entrez/query.fcgi?cmd=Retrieve&db=pubmed&dopt=Abstract&list_uids=15200237

- **Chronic (-)-hydroxycitrate administration spares carbohydrate utilization and promotes lipid oxidation during exercise in mice.**
  Author(s): Ishihara K, Oyaizu S, Onuki K, Lim K, Fushiki T.
  Source: The Journal of Nutrition. 2000 December; 130(12): 2990-5.
  http://www.ncbi.nlm.nih.gov/entrez/query.fcgi?cmd=Retrieve&db=pubmed&dopt=Abstract&list_uids=11110858

- **Dietary fat intake, supplements, and weight loss.**
  Author(s): Dyck DJ.
  Source: Canadian Journal of Applied Physiology = Revue Canadienne De Physiologie Appliquee. 2000 December; 25(6): 495-523. Review.
  http://www.ncbi.nlm.nih.gov/entrez/query.fcgi?cmd=Retrieve&db=pubmed&dopt=Abstract&list_uids=11187927

- **Effect of Garcinia cambogia extract on serum leptin and insulin in mice.**
  Author(s): Hayamizu K, Hirakawa H, Oikawa D, Nakanishi T, Takagi T, Tachibana T, Furuse M.
  Source: Fitoterapia. 2003 April; 74(3): 267-73.
  http://www.ncbi.nlm.nih.gov/entrez/query.fcgi?cmd=Retrieve&db=pubmed&dopt=Abstract&list_uids=12727492

- **Effect of hydroxycitric acid on serotonin release from isolated rat brain cortex.**
  Author(s): Ohia SE, Awe SO, LeDay AM, Opere CA, Bagchi D.
  Source: Res Commun Mol Pathol Pharmacol. 2001 March-April; 109(3-4): 210-6.
  http://www.ncbi.nlm.nih.gov/entrez/query.fcgi?cmd=Retrieve&db=pubmed&dopt=Abstract&list_uids=11758650

- **Effects of a natural extract of (-)-hydroxycitric acid (HCA-SX) and a combination of HCA-SX plus niacin-bound chromium and Gymnema sylvestre extract on weight loss.**
  Author(s): Preuss HG, Bagchi D, Bagchi M, Rao CV, Dey DK, Satyanarayana S.
  Source: Diabetes, Obesity & Metabolism. 2004 May; 6(3): 171-80.
  http://www.ncbi.nlm.nih.gov/entrez/query.fcgi?cmd=Retrieve&db=pubmed&dopt=Abstract&list_uids=15056124

- **Effects of niacin-bound chromium, Maitake mushroom fraction SX and (-)-hydroxycitric acid on the metabolic syndrome in aged diabetic Zucker fatty rats.**
  Author(s): Talpur N, Echard BW, Yasmin T, Bagchi D, Preuss HG.
  Source: Molecular and Cellular Biochemistry. 2003 October; 252(1-2): 369-77.
  http://www.ncbi.nlm.nih.gov/entrez/query.fcgi?cmd=Retrieve&db=pubmed&dopt=Abstract&list_uids=14577612

- **Garcinia cambogia (hydroxycitric acid) as a potential antiobesity agent: a randomized controlled trial.**
  Author(s): Heymsfield SB, Allison DB, Vasselli JR, Pietrobelli A, Greenfield D, Nunez C.
  Source: Jama : the Journal of the American Medical Association. 1998 November 11; 280(18): 1596-600.
  http://www.ncbi.nlm.nih.gov/entrez/query.fcgi?cmd=Retrieve&db=pubmed&dopt=Abstract&list_uids=9820262

- **In vitro and in vivo evaluation of potential aluminum chelators.**
  Author(s): Graff L, Muller G, Burnel D.
  Source: Vet Hum Toxicol. 1995 October; 37(5): 455-61.
  http://www.ncbi.nlm.nih.gov/entrez/query.fcgi?cmd=Retrieve&db=pubmed&dopt=Abstract&list_uids=8592836

- **Rhabdomyolysis in response to weight-loss herbal medicine.**
  Author(s): Mansi IA, Huang J.
  Source: The American Journal of the Medical Sciences. 2004 June; 327(6): 356-7.
  http://www.ncbi.nlm.nih.gov/entrez/query.fcgi?cmd=Retrieve&db=pubmed&dopt=Abstract&list_uids=15201651

- **Safety and mechanism of appetite suppression by a novel hydroxycitric acid extract (HCA-SX).**
  Author(s): Ohia SE, Opere CA, LeDay AM, Bagchi M, Bagchi D, Stohs SJ.
  Source: Molecular and Cellular Biochemistry. 2002 September; 238(1-2): 89-103.
  http://www.ncbi.nlm.nih.gov/entrez/query.fcgi?cmd=Retrieve&db=pubmed&dopt=Abstract&list_uids=12349913

- **Seizure activity and unresponsiveness after hydroxycut ingestion.**
  Author(s): Kockler DR, McCarthy MW, Lawson CL.
  Source: Pharmacotherapy. 2001 May; 21(5): 647-51.
  http://www.ncbi.nlm.nih.gov/entrez/query.fcgi?cmd=Retrieve&db=pubmed&dopt=Abstract&list_uids=11349754

- **Stimulation of islet protein kinase C translocation by palmitate requires metabolism of the fatty acid.**
  Author(s): Alcazar O, Qiu-yue Z, Gine E, Tamarit-Rodriguez J.
  Source: Diabetes. 1997 July; 46(7): 1153-8.
  http://www.ncbi.nlm.nih.gov/entrez/query.fcgi?cmd=Retrieve&db=pubmed&dopt=Abstract&list_uids=9200650

- **Supplemental products used for weight loss.**
  Author(s): Lenz TL, Hamilton WR.
  Source: J Am Pharm Assoc (Wash Dc). 2004 January-February; 44(1): 59-67; Quiz 67-8. Review.
  http://www.ncbi.nlm.nih.gov/entrez/query.fcgi?cmd=Retrieve&db=pubmed&dopt=Abstract&list_uids=14965155

Additional Web Resources

A number of additional Web sites offer encyclopedic information covering CAM and related topics. The following is a representative sample:

- Alternative Medicine Foundation, Inc.: http://www.herbmed.org/
- AOL: http://search.aol.com/cat.adp?id=169&layer=&from=subcats
- Chinese Medicine: http://www.newcenturynutrition.com/
- drkoop.com®: http://www.drkoop.com/InteractiveMedicine/IndexC.html
- Family Village: http://www.familyvillage.wisc.edu/med_altn.htm
- Google: http://directory.google.com/Top/Health/Alternative/
- Healthnotes: http://www.healthnotes.com/
- MedWebPlus: http://medwebplus.com/subject/Alternative_and_Complementary_Medicine
- Open Directory Project: http://dmoz.org/Health/Alternative/
- HealthGate: http://www.tnp.com/
- WebMD®Health: http://my.webmd.com/drugs_and_herbs
- WholeHealthMD.com: http://www.wholehealthmd.com/reflib/0,1529,00.html
- Yahoo.com: http://dir.yahoo.com/Health/Alternative_Medicine/

The following is a specific Web list relating to hydroxycitric acid; please note that any particular subject below may indicate either a therapeutic use, or a contraindication (potential danger), and does not reflect an official recommendation:

- General Overview

    Obesity
    Source: Integrative Medicine Communications; www.drkoop.com

    Weight Loss and Obesity
    Source: Healthnotes, Inc.; www.healthnotes.com

- Herbs and Supplements

    Garcinia Cambogia
    Alternative names: Citrin, Gambooge
    Source: Alternative Medicine Foundation, Inc.; www.amfoundation.org

    Hibiscus
    Alternative names: Hibiscus, Roselle; Hibiscus sp.
    Source: Alternative Medicine Foundation, Inc.; www.amfoundation.org

    Hydroxycitric Acid
    Source: Healthnotes, Inc.; www.healthnotes.com

Hydroxycitric Acid
Source: Prima Communications, Inc. www.personalhealthzone.com

General References

A good place to find general background information on CAM is the National Library of Medicine. It has prepared within the MEDLINEplus system an information topic page dedicated to complementary and alternative medicine. To access this page, go to the MEDLINEplus site at **http://www.nlm.nih.gov/medlineplus/alternativemedicine.html**. This Web site provides a general overview of various topics and can lead to a number of general sources.

CHAPTER 4. PATENTS ON HYDROXYCITRIC ACID

Overview

Patents can be physical innovations (e.g. chemicals, pharmaceuticals, medical equipment) or processes (e.g. treatments or diagnostic procedures). The United States Patent and Trademark Office defines a patent as a grant of a property right to the inventor, issued by the Patent and Trademark Office.[5] Patents, therefore, are intellectual property. For the United States, the term of a new patent is 20 years from the date when the patent application was filed. If the inventor wishes to receive economic benefits, it is likely that the invention will become commercially available within 20 years of the initial filing. It is important to understand, therefore, that an inventor's patent does not indicate that a product or service is or will be commercially available. The patent implies only that the inventor has "the right to exclude others from making, using, offering for sale, or selling" the invention in the United States. While this relates to U.S. patents, similar rules govern foreign patents.

In this chapter, we show you how to locate information on patents and their inventors. If you find a patent that is particularly interesting to you, contact the inventor or the assignee for further information. **IMPORTANT NOTE:** When following the search strategy described below, you may discover <u>non-medical patents</u> that use the generic term "hydroxycitric acid" (or a synonym) in their titles. To accurately reflect the results that you might find while conducting research on hydroxycitric acid, <u>we have not necessarily excluded non-medical patents</u> in this bibliography.

Patents on Hydroxycitric Acid

By performing a patent search focusing on hydroxycitric acid, you can obtain information such as the title of the invention, the names of the inventor(s), the assignee(s) or the company that owns or controls the patent, a short abstract that summarizes the patent, and a few excerpts from the description of the patent. The abstract of a patent tends to be more technical in nature, while the description is often written for the public. Full patent descriptions contain much more information than is presented here (e.g. claims, references, figures, diagrams, etc.). We will tell you how to obtain this information later in the chapter.

---

[5]Adapted from the United States Patent and Trademark Office: http://www.uspto.gov/web/offices/pac/doc/general/whatis.htm.

The following is an example of the type of information that you can expect to obtain from a patent search on hydroxycitric acid:

- **Convenient method for large-scale isolation of hibiscus acid**

    Inventor(s): Ibnusaud; Ibrahim (Kottayam, IN), Philip; Teena (Kottayam, IN), Rajasekharan; Rani (Kottayam, IN), Thomas; Salini (Kottayam, IN)

    Assignee(s): Department of Science and Technology, Goverment of India (IN)

    Patent Number: 6,127,553

    Date filed: July 30, 1999

    Abstract: The invention relates to a process for the isolation of Hibiscus acid or (+)hydroxycitric acid lactone (2S,3R-dihydroxy-1,2,3-propanetricarboxylic acid lactone) from the leaves of Hibiscus furcatus, Hibiscus sabdariffa and Hibiscus cannabinus. Garcinia acid, one of the optical isomers of **hydroxycitric acid** is a potentially interesting molecule and found extensive application in the pharmacological as well as synthetic fronts.

    Excerpt(s): 7. JCS Chem. Comm. pp. 711, 1973). However only very little information is available on Hibiscus acid (Ia), another optical isomer of hydroxy citric acid. The potential of the molecule is not yet explored due to the non-availability of the compound in the market. There is no economically viable large-scale isolation procedure available for this compound. Though Y. S. Lewis & S. Neelakantan (Phytochemistry. vol 4, pp 619-624, 1965) describes the presence of hibiscus acid in the leaves of Hibiscus furcatus and Hibiscus cannabinus, no method is reported on the isolation of the acid in large scale. Hence the present invention assumes importance. a. The method reported by Per. M. Boll, Else Sorensen and Erik Balieu (Acta Chem. Scand 23 pp. 286-293, 1969) for the isolation of Hibiscus acid is from the calyx of the fruits of Hibiscus sabdariffa. In this method dried, ground calyxes of Hibiscus sabdariffa fruits are extracted at room temperature for 68 hours several times with methanol containing 1.5% hydrogen chloride. To the pooled methanol extracts, ether is added and the coloring matter is deposited as a dark red syrupy mass. Ether layer is collected and syrup is dissolved in methanolic hydrogen chloride (1%) and again precipitated by the addition of ether. The pooled ether extracts are evaporated and is dissolved in methanol. Upon cooling colorless crystals are obtained and the same is recrystallised from propanol.

    Web site: http://www.delphion.com/details?pn=US06127553__

- **Hydroxycitric acid concentrate and food products prepared therefrom**

    Inventor(s): Balasubramanvam; Karanam (7971, 2nd Main, IIIrd Block, Thyagaraja Nagar, Bangalore, IN), Bhandari; Ashok Kumar (2/4A Kensington Road, Bangalore, IN), Moffett; Scott Alexander (12730 Mulholland Dr., Beverly Hills, CA 90210), Ravindranath; Bhagavathula (714, 7th Main Road, J. P. Nagar III phase, Bangalore, IN)

    Assignee(s): none reported

    Patent Number: 5,656,314

    Date filed: April 17, 1996

    Abstract: A **hydroxycitric acid** concentrate prepared from Garcinia rind including 23 to 54% by weight free **hydroxycitric acid,** 6 to 20% by weight lactone of **hydroxycitric acid,** 0.001 to 8% by weight citric acid, and 32 to 70% by weight water, wherein the free

hydroxycitric acid, the lactone of **hydroxycitric acid** and the citric acid constitute 94 to 99% by weight of total solutes dissolved in the water. Also disclosed is a method of preparing such a concentrate from Garcinia rind, as well as food products containing **hydroxycitric acid**.

Excerpt(s): Hydroxycitric acid, both free acid and lactone forms, is present in the fruit rind, of Garcinia species (e.g., Garcinia cambogia, Garcinia atroviridis, and Garcinia indica), which are commercially available in India. As an inhibitor of the synthesis of fat and cholesterol, **hydroxycitric acid** has been shown to significantly reduce the body weight and lower lipid accumulation in rats. See, e.g., Sergio, W., Medical Hypothesis 27: 39 (1988); and Sullivan, A. C. et al., Lipids 9: 121 (1973); and Sullivan, A. C. et al., Lipids 9: 129 (1973). **Hydroxycitric acid** is also the only known anorectic agent found as a natural constituent of edible foods consumed by humans. Methods for the extraction and purification of **hydroxycitric acid** from Garcinia rind can be found in Lewis, Y. S., Methods in Enzymology 13: 613 (1967); and Indian Patent No. 160753.

Web site: http://www.delphion.com/details?pn=US05656314__

- **Soluble double metal salt of group IA and IIA of (-) hydroxycitric acid, process of preparing the same and its use in beverages and other food products without effecting their flavor and properties**

   Inventor(s): Balasubramanyam; Karanam (Bangalore, IN), Chandrasekhar; Bhaskaran (Bangalore, IN), Ramadoss; Candadai Seshadri (Bangalore, IN), Rao; Pillarisetti Venkata Subba (Bangalore, IN)

   Assignee(s): Vittal Mallya Scientific Research Foundation (Bangalore, IN)

   Patent Number: 6,160,172

   Date filed: April 14, 1998

   Abstract: The present invention is directed to a new soluble double metal salt of group IA and IIA of (-) **hydroxycitric acid** of general formula I:where X is IA group metal: Li or Na or K or Rb or Cs or Frwhere Y is IIA group metal: Be or Mg or Ca or Sr or Ba or Rawhere the concentration of X in the salt varies from 1.5-51.0%,the concentration of Y in the salts varies from 2.0-50.9%,the concentration of HCA in the salt varies from 31.0-93.0% depending on the nature of X and Y.This invention more particularly relates to new soluble double metal salt of group IA and IIA of (-) **hydroxycitric acid** of general formula II.This invention also includes a process of preparing the soluble double metal salt of group IA and IIA of (-) **hydroxycitric acid** of general formula I comprising: preparing (-) **hydroxycitric acid** liquid concentrate/solid lactone of hyroxycitric acid from Garcinia extract, neutralizing the free (-) **hydroxycitric acid** present in the said (-) **hydroxycitric acid** liquid concentrate/solid lactone (-) **hydroxycitric acid** with group IA metal hydroxides, displacing partially the group IA metal ions in the above salt solutions by adding group IIA metal chlorides to form soluble double metal salt of group IA and IIA of (-) **hydroxycitric acid**, precipitating the said double metal salt of group IA & IIA of (-) **hydroxycitric acid** by adding aqueous polar solvent to get soluble IIA metal salt of (-) **hydroxycitric acid** or obtaining the soluble double metal salt as powder by spray drying prior to the solvent addition or spray drying water solubilised solvent precipitated material.The instant invention also discloses the use of the said soluble double metal salt of group IA and IIA of (-) **hydroxycitric acid** of formula I and particularly formula II in beverages and other food products and its use in beverages and other food products.

Excerpt(s): This invention relates to a new soluble double metal salt of group IA and II A of (-) **hydroxycitric acid,** process of preparing the same and its use in beverages and other food products without effecting their flavor and properties. This product with >98% purity can be used safely not only as a food supplement in various nutriceutical formulations and beverages but also for effecting obesity control. (-) **Hydroxycitric acid** HCA) occurs in the fruit rind of Garcinia species (G. Cambogia, G. indica and G. atroviridis). The first two species grow abundantly in India and the third occurs mostly in South East Asian countries. The success of this natural food product derived from Garcinia fruit has been documented and been in use since several centuries BC. Also known as "Kokum", the extracts of the fruit have been used as a tart flavoring in meat and seafood dishes, turned into a refreshing beverage that serves as a unique flavor enhancer, gourmet spice and a digestive after a heavy meal. In Ayurveda, the traditional ancient system of herbal medicine in India, Garcinia is also considered to be one of the prime herbs that are beneficial for the heart. In more recent times, Garcinia has received worldwide attention as a nutriceutical for effective obesity control. Several scientists including at Hoffman-La Roche have established that HCA, the active ingredient in the fruit, prevents the conversion of excess carbohydrates to fat in animals. The energy released by the excess carbohydrate is converted into and stored as glycogen, a readily usable form of energy. Interestingly, it has been shown to inhibit ATP dependent citrate-lyase, a key enzyme in diverting carbohydrate to fatty acids and cholesterol synthesis (Sullivan et al. Lipids, 9:121 and 129 (1973), Sergio, W., Medical Hypotehsis 27:39 (1988)).

Web site: http://www.delphion.com/details?pn=US06160172__

- **Weight control product and method of treating hyperlipidemia and increasing vigor with said product**

Inventor(s): Brink; William DesIsles (Newton, MA)

Assignee(s): Prolab Nutrition, Inc. (Bloomfield, CT)

Patent Number: 6,113,949

Date filed: October 27, 1998

Abstract: This invention relates to a weight control composition, preferably in the form of a capsule or tablet, comprising a mixture of guggul extract and at least one phosphate salt selected from calcium phosphate, potassium phosphate and sodium phosphate. The composition evidences synergistic activity in reducing body weight and percent body fat in mammals. The guggul extract/phosphate salt product also reduces plasma lipid levels and cholesterol in overweight hyperlipidaemic humans. The inventive composition may also contain at least one additional component selected from phosphatidylcholine, **hydroxycitric acid** and L-tyrosine.

Excerpt(s): This invention relates generally to a weight control product that is administered enterally to mammals in need of losing weight and/or reducing the blood plasma lipid levels. The weight control product comprises a mixture of guggul extract and phosphate salts. The inventive product is also useful in enhancing mood states, increasing vigor and reducing blood serum lipid levels. The weight control product of the present invention is designed to promote weight loss as a component of a weight control program for individuals who are overweight and desire to lose body fat and/or reduce their plasma lipid levels. The product according to the invention is consumed as a nutritional supplement and is preferably incorporated into a multi-disciplinary nutritional program such as the American Heart Association Step One Diet. Numerous weight control products are known in the literature. One example of a weight control product is taught in U.S. Pat. No. 4,959,227 to Amer wherein the product has a reduced lactose content and contains dietary fiber. In similar fashion, U.S. Pat. No. 5,104,676 to Mahmoud et al. discloses a weight loss product that utilizes a particular blend of soluble, insoluble, fermentable and non-fermentable fibers. Commercially available weight control products include Ultra-Slim Fast.RTM. which is distributed by Slim Fast Foods, a division of Thompson Medical Company, Inc. New York, N.Y. and OpitiTrim.RTM. which is available from the Clinical Products Division of Sandoz Nutrition Corp., Minneapolis, Minn. In addition, literally hundreds of chemical entities have been suggested as weight loss products, however, none of the prior art has suggested or disclosed the combined use of a guggul extract with a blend of phosphate salts to result in a composition that is highly effective in reducing the weight of a mammal through primarily a loss of body fat while at the same time dramatically decreasing the blood plasma lipid levels of the individual, enhancing the mood states and increasing vigor.

Web site: http://www.delphion.com/details?pn=US06113949__

Patent Applications on Hydroxycitric Acid

As of December 2000, U.S. patent applications are open to public viewing.[6] Applications are patent requests which have yet to be granted. (The process to achieve a patent can take several years.) The following patent applications have been filed since December 2000 relating to hydroxycitric acid:

- **Bioavailable composition of natural and synthetic hca**

    Inventor(s): Hadmaev, Vladimir; (Piscataway, NJ), Majeed, Muhammed; (Piscataway, NJ)

    Correspondence: Arent Fox Kintner Plotkin & Kahn; 1050 Connecticut Avenue, N.W.; Suite 400; Washington; DC; 20036; US

    Patent Application Number: 20020187943

    Date filed: June 6, 2002

    Abstract: The invention relates to a composition comprising **hydroxycitric acid** (HCA) in combination with either one or both of garcinol and anthocyanin, and its use as a weight-loss therapy in animal subjects, preferably humans. The therapeutic effects for the composition observed in murine and human studies include a reduction in total body weight and body mass index, a reduction in body fat, an increase in lean body mass and content of body water, and a reduction in perceived appetite level. Another composition for use in weight-loss therapy is also described relating to forskolin in combination with either one or both of garcinol and anthocyanin. The anti-oxidant properties of garcinol are described as being enhanced in the presence of HCA and anthocyanin, and the combination of HCA, garcinol and anthocyanin is also shown to exert greater citrate lyase inhibiting properties than either compound alone. Methods of obtaining HCA, garcinol or anthocyanin, or a composition containing all three compounds, are described.

    Excerpt(s): This application claims priority under 35 U.S.C.sctn. 1.119(e) to provisional application serial No. 60/225,821, filed on Aug. 17, 2000. Although the potential of (-

---

[6] This has been a common practice outside the United States prior to December 2000.

)HCA as a weight lowering compound has been recognized since the 1970's, only few clinical studies have been conducted with this compound. (7-12). These few studies examining HCA-mediated prevention of excess body fat, resulted in contradictory results, most likely due to HCA being poorly bioavailable in the cytosol of a target cell. In one clinical study of HCA, a controversial high fiber diet was used. The use of a high-fiber diet in combination with HCA may reduce gastrointestinal absorption of HCA, since high-fiber diets are known to reduce absorption of many nutrients and micronutrients. This issue becomes critical with HCA because its reported efficacy in inhibiting the intracellular enzyme, adenosine triphosphate (ATP)-citrate-lyase, depends entirely on the presence of HCA inside the target cell. In their U.S. Patent, the Inventors addressed an important issue regarding the bioavailability of the HCA compounds. The U.S. Pat. No. 5,783,603 patent described a manufacturing process leading to a unique structure for a potassium salt of HCA, which facilitated its transport across biological membranes, effectively delivering more HCA into the cytosol for the competitive inhibition of ATP citrate lyase. Although the '603 patent related to an HCA compound having considerably improved bioavailability, its bioavailability was still relatively inefficient. For example, an in vitro study done on hepatic cells, indicates that 5 mM of extracellular potassium HCA could inhibit ATP citrate lyase. However, only 0.5 mM of potassium HCA is actually needed in the cytosol to effectively inhibit ATP citrate lyase. Therefore, a 10-fold excess amount of potassium HCA is needed outside of the target cell in order to achieve a concentration of {fraction (1/10)} that amount in the cytosol. This finding of relatively poor bioavailability of HCA, was confirmed in pre-clinical experiments (14), and points out the need to further improve the bioavailability and efficacy of HCA.

Web site: http://appft1.uspto.gov/netahtml/PTO/search-bool.html

- **Compositions incorporating(-)-hydroxycitric acid, chromium, and gymnemic acid, and related methods for promoting healthy body weight and improving related health factors**

    Inventor(s): Bagchi, Debasis; (Concord, CA), Preuss, Harry G.; (Fairfax Station, VA)

    Correspondence: Sheppard, Mullin, Richter & Hampton Llp; 333 South Hope Street; 48th Floor; Los Angeles; CA; 90071-1448; US

    Patent Application Number: 20040014692

    Date filed: December 20, 2002

    Abstract: Methods for promoting healthy body weight and improving a variety of related physiological factors, including serum serotonin levels, serum leptin levels, fat oxidation, cholesterol levels, and body mass index, in persons or other mammals, include administering to those persons or other mammals effective amounts of **hydroxycitric acid** or a combination of **hydroxycitric acid**, chromium and gymnemic acid, which work synergistically to further to promote healthy body weight and improve these physiological factors.

    Excerpt(s): This application claims the benefit of U.S. Provisional Patent Application Serial No. 60/343,473, filed Dec. 20, 2001. The present invention relates generally to compositions and related methods for promoting healthy body weight, including reducing excess body weight or maintaining healthy body weight, and improving related health factors, such as cholesterol levels and body mass index, in persons and other mammals. Excess body weight is becoming more prevalent worldwide at an alarming rate, both in developing and developed countries. Approximately 61 percent of adults in the U.S. are overweight (i.e., having a body mass index (BMI) of greater than 25 kg/m.sup.2), while more than 26 percent of U.S. adults are obese (i.e., having a BMI of greater than 30 kg/m.sup.2). Obesity is the second leading cause of premature death in the U.S. Approximately 300,000 Americans die each year from complications caused by obesity. According to the World Health Organization, there are over 300 million obese adults worldwide. Environmental and behavioral changes brought about by economic development, modernization and urbanization have been linked to the global rise in obesity in adults and children, the true health consequences of which may not be fully known for years to come. Consumption of western-style diets, low levels of physical activity and sedentary lifestyles generally have been implicated in the worldwide trend of weight gain.

Web site: http://appft1.uspto.gov/netahtml/PTO/search-bool.html

- **Hydroxycitric acid salt composition and method of making**

    Inventor(s): Bhaskaran, Sunil; (Wanorie, IN), Mehta, Sevanti; (Houston, TX)

    Correspondence: Conley Rose, P.C.; P. O. Box 3267; Houston; TX; 77253-3267; US

    Patent Application Number: 20030207942

    Date filed: April 29, 2003

    Abstract: Disclosed is a **hydroxycitric acid** salt composition comprising calcium and potassium salts of **hydroxycitric acid**, preferably in a defined proportion which yields a very pure, stabilized preparation that is substantially tasteless for optimal use in a variety of foods items. The HCA salts are prepared by a process that includes treating an aqueous extract of Garcinia cambogia or Garcinia indica fruit with a liquid quaternizing agent such as a trialkylamine in which the alkyl groups are octyl, caprylyl, isooctyl, lauryl or decyl.

    Excerpt(s): This application claims the benefit under 35 U.S.C.sctn.119(e) of U.S. Provisional Patent Application No. 60/376,490 filed Apr. 30, 2002, the disclosure of which is hereby incorporated herein by reference. Not applicable. The present invention generally relates to **hydroxycitric acid** (HCA) and its salts, and more specifically to water soluble mixtures of calcium and potassium salts of HCA, and to methods of making the calcium and potassium salts and mixtures thereof. The invention also relates to the use of such compositions as nutraceuticals or dietary supplements.

    Web site: http://appft1.uspto.gov/netahtml/PTO/search-bool.html

Keeping Current

In order to stay informed about patents and patent applications dealing with hydroxycitric acid, you can access the U.S. Patent Office archive via the Internet at the following Web address: **http://www.uspto.gov/patft/index.html**. You will see two broad options: (1) Issued Patent, and (2) Published Applications. To see a list of issued patents, perform the following steps: Under "Issued Patents," click "Quick Search." Then, type "hydroxycitric acid" (or synonyms) into the "Term 1" box. After clicking on the search button, scroll down to see the various patents which have been granted to date on hydroxycitric acid.

You can also use this procedure to view pending patent applications concerning hydroxycitric acid. Simply go back to **http://www.uspto.gov/patft/index.html**. Select "Quick Search" under "Published Applications." Then proceed with the steps listed above.

APPENDICES

APPENDIX A. PHYSICIAN RESOURCES

Overview

In this chapter, we focus on databases and Internet-based guidelines and information resources created or written for a professional audience.

NIH Guidelines

Commonly referred to as "clinical" or "professional" guidelines, the National Institutes of Health publish physician guidelines for the most common diseases. Publications are available at the following by relevant Institute[7]:

- Office of the Director (OD); guidelines consolidated across agencies available at
  http://www.nih.gov/health/consumer/conkey.htm

- National Institute of General Medical Sciences (NIGMS); fact sheets available at
  http://www.nigms.nih.gov/news/facts/

- National Library of Medicine (NLM); extensive encyclopedia (A.D.A.M., Inc.) with guidelines: http://www.nlm.nih.gov/medlineplus/healthtopics.html

- National Cancer Institute (NCI); guidelines available at
  http://www.cancer.gov/cancerinfo/list.aspx?viewid=5f35036e-5497-4d86-8c2c-714a9f7c8d25

- National Eye Institute (NEI); guidelines available at
  http://www.nei.nih.gov/order/index.htm

- National Heart, Lung, and Blood Institute (NHLBI); guidelines available at
  http://www.nhlbi.nih.gov/guidelines/index.htm

- National Human Genome Research Institute (NHGRI); research available at
  http://www.genome.gov/page.cfm?pageID=10000375

- National Institute on Aging (NIA); guidelines available at
  http://www.nia.nih.gov/health/

---

[7] These publications are typically written by one or more of the various NIH Institutes.

- National Institute on Alcohol Abuse and Alcoholism (NIAAA); guidelines available at http://www.niaaa.nih.gov/publications/publications.htm
- National Institute of Allergy and Infectious Diseases (NIAID); guidelines available at http://www.niaid.nih.gov/publications/
- National Institute of Arthritis and Musculoskeletal and Skin Diseases (NIAMS); fact sheets and guidelines available at http://www.niams.nih.gov/hi/index.htm
- National Institute of Child Health and Human Development (NICHD); guidelines available at http://www.nichd.nih.gov/publications/pubskey.cfm
- National Institute on Deafness and Other Communication Disorders (NIDCD); fact sheets and guidelines at http://www.nidcd.nih.gov/health/
- National Institute of Dental and Craniofacial Research (NIDCR); guidelines available at http://www.nidr.nih.gov/health/
- National Institute of Diabetes and Digestive and Kidney Diseases (NIDDK); guidelines available at http://www.niddk.nih.gov/health/health.htm
- National Institute on Drug Abuse (NIDA); guidelines available at http://www.nida.nih.gov/DrugAbuse.html
- National Institute of Environmental Health Sciences (NIEHS); environmental health information available at http://www.niehs.nih.gov/external/facts.htm
- National Institute of Mental Health (NIMH); guidelines available at http://www.nimh.nih.gov/practitioners/index.cfm
- National Institute of Neurological Disorders and Stroke (NINDS); neurological disorder information pages available at http://www.ninds.nih.gov/health_and_medical/disorder_index.htm
- National Institute of Nursing Research (NINR); publications on selected illnesses at http://www.nih.gov/ninr/news-info/publications.html
- National Institute of Biomedical Imaging and Bioengineering; general information at http://grants.nih.gov/grants/becon/becon_info.htm
- Center for Information Technology (CIT); referrals to other agencies based on keyword searches available at http://kb.nih.gov/www_query_main.asp
- National Center for Complementary and Alternative Medicine (NCCAM); health information available at http://nccam.nih.gov/health/
- National Center for Research Resources (NCRR); various information directories available at http://www.ncrr.nih.gov/publications.asp
- Office of Rare Diseases; various fact sheets available at http://rarediseases.info.nih.gov/html/resources/rep_pubs.html
- Centers for Disease Control and Prevention; various fact sheets on infectious diseases available at http://www.cdc.gov/publications.htm

NIH Databases

In addition to the various Institutes of Health that publish professional guidelines, the NIH has designed a number of databases for professionals.[8] Physician-oriented resources provide a wide variety of information related to the biomedical and health sciences, both past and present. The format of these resources varies. Searchable databases, bibliographic citations, full-text articles (when available), archival collections, and images are all available. The following are referenced by the National Library of Medicine:[9]

- **Bioethics:** Access to published literature on the ethical, legal, and public policy issues surrounding healthcare and biomedical research. This information is provided in conjunction with the Kennedy Institute of Ethics located at Georgetown University, Washington, D.C.: http://www.nlm.nih.gov/databases/databases_bioethics.html

- **HIV/AIDS Resources:** Describes various links and databases dedicated to HIV/AIDS research: http://www.nlm.nih.gov/pubs/factsheets/aidsinfs.html

- **NLM Online Exhibitions:** Describes "Exhibitions in the History of Medicine": http://www.nlm.nih.gov/exhibition/exhibition.html. Additional resources for historical scholarship in medicine: http://www.nlm.nih.gov/hmd/hmd.html

- **Biotechnology Information:** Access to public databases. The National Center for Biotechnology Information conducts research in computational biology, develops software tools for analyzing genome data, and disseminates biomedical information for the better understanding of molecular processes affecting human health and disease: http://www.ncbi.nlm.nih.gov/

- **Population Information:** The National Library of Medicine provides access to worldwide coverage of population, family planning, and related health issues, including family planning technology and programs, fertility, and population law and policy: http://www.nlm.nih.gov/databases/databases_population.html

- **Cancer Information:** Access to cancer-oriented databases: http://www.nlm.nih.gov/databases/databases_cancer.html

- **Profiles in Science:** Offering the archival collections of prominent twentieth-century biomedical scientists to the public through modern digital technology: http://www.profiles.nlm.nih.gov/

- **Chemical Information:** Provides links to various chemical databases and references: http://sis.nlm.nih.gov/Chem/ChemMain.html

- **Clinical Alerts:** Reports the release of findings from the NIH-funded clinical trials where such release could significantly affect morbidity and mortality: http://www.nlm.nih.gov/databases/alerts/clinical_alerts.html

- **Space Life Sciences:** Provides links and information to space-based research (including NASA): http://www.nlm.nih.gov/databases/databases_space.html

- **MEDLINE:** Bibliographic database covering the fields of medicine, nursing, dentistry, veterinary medicine, the healthcare system, and the pre-clinical sciences: http://www.nlm.nih.gov/databases/databases_medline.html

---

[8] Remember, for the general public, the National Library of Medicine recommends the databases referenced in MEDLINE*plus* (http://medlineplus.gov/ or http://www.nlm.nih.gov/medlineplus/databases.html).

[9] See http://www.nlm.nih.gov/databases/databases.html.

- **Toxicology and Environmental Health Information (TOXNET):** Databases covering toxicology and environmental health: http://sis.nlm.nih.gov/Tox/ToxMain.html

- **Visible Human Interface:** Anatomically detailed, three-dimensional representations of normal male and female human bodies:
http://www.nlm.nih.gov/research/visible/visible_human.html

The NLM Gateway[10]

The NLM (National Library of Medicine) Gateway is a Web-based system that lets users search simultaneously in multiple retrieval systems at the U.S. National Library of Medicine (NLM). It allows users of NLM services to initiate searches from one Web interface, providing one-stop searching for many of NLM's information resources or databases.[11] To use the NLM Gateway, simply go to the search site at **http://gateway.nlm.nih.gov/gw/Cmd**. Type "hydroxycitric acid" (or synonyms) into the search box and click "Search." The results will be presented in a tabular form, indicating the number of references in each database category.

Results Summary

Category	Items Found
Journal Articles	94
Books / Periodicals / Audio Visual	0
Consumer Health	0
Meeting Abstracts	0
Other Collections	7833
Total	7927

HSTAT[12]

HSTAT is a free, Web-based resource that provides access to full-text documents used in healthcare decision-making.[13] These documents include clinical practice guidelines, quick-reference guides for clinicians, consumer health brochures, evidence reports and technology assessments from the Agency for Healthcare Research and Quality (AHRQ), as well as AHRQ's Put Prevention Into Practice.[14] Simply search by "hydroxycitric acid" (or synonyms) at the following Web site: **http://text.nlm.nih.gov**.

---

[10] Adapted from NLM: http://gateway.nlm.nih.gov/gw/Cmd?Overview.x.

[11] The NLM Gateway is currently being developed by the Lister Hill National Center for Biomedical Communications (LHNCBC) at the National Library of Medicine (NLM) of the National Institutes of Health (NIH).

[12] Adapted from HSTAT: http://www.nlm.nih.gov/pubs/factsheets/hstat.html.

[13] The HSTAT URL is http://hstat.nlm.nih.gov/.

[14] Other important documents in HSTAT include: the National Institutes of Health (NIH) Consensus Conference Reports and Technology Assessment Reports; the HIV/AIDS Treatment Information Service (ATIS) resource documents; the Substance Abuse and Mental Health Services Administration's Center for Substance Abuse Treatment (SAMHSA/CSAT) Treatment Improvement Protocols (TIP) and Center for Substance Abuse Prevention (SAMHSA/CSAP) Prevention Enhancement Protocols System (PEPS); the Public Health Service (PHS) Preventive Services Task Force's *Guide to Clinical Preventive Services*; the independent, nonfederal Task Force on Community Services' *Guide to Community Preventive Services*; and the Health Technology Advisory Committee (HTAC) of the Minnesota Health Care Commission (MHCC) health technology evaluations.

Coffee Break: Tutorials for Biologists[15]

Coffee Break is a general healthcare site that takes a scientific view of the news and covers recent breakthroughs in biology that may one day assist physicians in developing treatments. Here you will find a collection of short reports on recent biological discoveries. Each report incorporates interactive tutorials that demonstrate how bioinformatics tools are used as a part of the research process. Currently, all Coffee Breaks are written by NCBI staff.[16] Each report is about 400 words and is usually based on a discovery reported in one or more articles from recently published, peer-reviewed literature.[17] This site has new articles every few weeks, so it can be considered an online magazine of sorts. It is intended for general background information. You can access the Coffee Break Web site at the following hyperlink: **http://www.ncbi.nlm.nih.gov/Coffeebreak/**.

Other Commercial Databases

In addition to resources maintained by official agencies, other databases exist that are commercial ventures addressing medical professionals. Here are some examples that may interest you:

- **CliniWeb International:** Index and table of contents to selected clinical information on the Internet; see **http://www.ohsu.edu/cliniweb/**.

- **Medical World Search:** Searches full text from thousands of selected medical sites on the Internet; see **http://www.mwsearch.com/**.

---

[15] Adapted from **http://www.ncbi.nlm.nih.gov/Coffeebreak/Archive/FAQ.html**.

[16] The figure that accompanies each article is frequently supplied by an expert external to NCBI, in which case the source of the figure is cited. The result is an interactive tutorial that tells a biological story.

[17] After a brief introduction that sets the work described into a broader context, the report focuses on how a molecular understanding can provide explanations of observed biology and lead to therapies for diseases. Each vignette is accompanied by a figure and hypertext links that lead to a series of pages that interactively show how NCBI tools and resources are used in the research process.

APPENDIX B. PATIENT RESOURCES

Overview

Official agencies, as well as federally funded institutions supported by national grants, frequently publish a variety of guidelines written with the patient in mind. These are typically called "Fact Sheets" or "Guidelines." They can take the form of a brochure, information kit, pamphlet, or flyer. Often they are only a few pages in length. Since new guidelines on hydroxycitric acid can appear at any moment and be published by a number of sources, the best approach to finding guidelines is to systematically scan the Internet-based services that post them.

Patient Guideline Sources

The remainder of this chapter directs you to sources which either publish or can help you find additional guidelines on topics related to hydroxycitric acid. Due to space limitations, these sources are listed in a concise manner. Do not hesitate to consult the following sources by either using the Internet hyperlink provided, or, in cases where the contact information is provided, contacting the publisher or author directly.

The National Institutes of Health

The NIH gateway to patients is located at **http://health.nih.gov/**. From this site, you can search across various sources and institutes, a number of which are summarized below.

Topic Pages: MEDLINEplus

The National Library of Medicine has created a vast and patient-oriented healthcare information portal called MEDLINEplus. Within this Internet-based system are "health topic pages" which list links to available materials relevant to hydroxycitric acid. To access this system, log on to **http://www.nlm.nih.gov/medlineplus/healthtopics.html**. From there you can either search using the alphabetical index or browse by broad topic areas. Recently, MEDLINEplus listed the following when searched for "hydroxycitric acid":

Herbal Medicine
http://www.nlm.nih.gov/medlineplus/herbalmedicine.html

Weight Loss and Dieting
http://www.nlm.nih.gov/medlineplus/weightlossanddieting.html

You may also choose to use the search utility provided by MEDLINEplus at the following Web address: **http://www.nlm.nih.gov/medlineplus/**. Simply type a keyword into the search box and click "Search." This utility is similar to the NIH search utility, with the exception that it only includes materials that are linked within the MEDLINEplus system (mostly patient-oriented information). It also has the disadvantage of generating unstructured results. We recommend, therefore, that you use this method only if you have a very targeted search.

The NIH Search Utility

The NIH search utility allows you to search for documents on over 100 selected Web sites that comprise the NIH-WEB-SPACE. Each of these servers is "crawled" and indexed on an ongoing basis. Your search will produce a list of various documents, all of which will relate in some way to hydroxycitric acid. The drawbacks of this approach are that the information is not organized by theme and that the references are often a mix of information for professionals and patients. Nevertheless, a large number of the listed Web sites provide useful background information. We can only recommend this route, therefore, for relatively rare or specific disorders, or when using highly targeted searches. To use the NIH search utility, visit the following Web page: **http://search.nih.gov/index.html**.

Additional Web Sources

A number of Web sites are available to the public that often link to government sites. These can also point you in the direction of essential information. The following is a representative sample:

- AOL: **http://search.aol.com/cat.adp?id=168&layer=&from=subcats**
- Family Village: **http://www.familyvillage.wisc.edu/specific.htm**
- Google: **http://directory.google.com/Top/Health/Conditions_and_Diseases/**
- Med Help International: **http://www.medhelp.org/HealthTopics/A.html**
- Open Directory Project: **http://dmoz.org/Health/Conditions_and_Diseases/**
- Yahoo.com: **http://dir.yahoo.com/Health/Diseases_and_Conditions/**
- WebMD®Health: **http://my.webmd.com/health_topics**

Finding Associations

There are several Internet directories that provide lists of medical associations with information on or resources relating to hydroxycitric acid. By consulting all of associations listed in this chapter, you will have nearly exhausted all sources for patient associations concerned with hydroxycitric acid.

The National Health Information Center (NHIC)

The National Health Information Center (NHIC) offers a free referral service to help people find organizations that provide information about hydroxycitric acid. For more information, see the NHIC's Web site at **http://www.health.gov/NHIC/** or contact an information specialist by calling 1-800-336-4797.

Directory of Health Organizations

The Directory of Health Organizations, provided by the National Library of Medicine Specialized Information Services, is a comprehensive source of information on associations. The Directory of Health Organizations database can be accessed via the Internet at **http://www.sis.nlm.nih.gov/Dir/DirMain.html**. It is composed of two parts: DIRLINE and Health Hotlines.

The DIRLINE database comprises some 10,000 records of organizations, research centers, and government institutes and associations that primarily focus on health and biomedicine. To access DIRLINE directly, go to the following Web site: **http://dirline.nlm.nih.gov/**. Simply type in "hydroxycitric acid" (or a synonym), and you will receive information on all relevant organizations listed in the database.

Health Hotlines directs you to toll-free numbers to over 300 organizations. You can access this database directly at **http://www.sis.nlm.nih.gov/hotlines/**. On this page, you are given the option to search by keyword or by browsing the subject list. When you have received your search results, click on the name of the organization for its description and contact information.

The Combined Health Information Database

Another comprehensive source of information on healthcare associations is the Combined Health Information Database. Using the "Detailed Search" option, you will need to limit your search to "Organizations" and "hydroxycitric acid". Type the following hyperlink into your Web browser: **http://chid.nih.gov/detail/detail.html**. To find associations, use the drop boxes at the bottom of the search page where "You may refine your search by." For publication date, select "All Years." Then, select your preferred language and the format option "Organization Resource Sheet." Type "hydroxycitric acid" (or synonyms) into the "For these words:" box. You should check back periodically with this database since it is updated every three months.

The National Organization for Rare Disorders, Inc.

The National Organization for Rare Disorders, Inc. has prepared a Web site that provides, at no charge, lists of associations organized by health topic. You can access this database at the following Web site: **http://www.rarediseases.org/search/orgsearch.html**. Type "hydroxycitric acid" (or a synonym) into the search box, and click "Submit Query."

APPENDIX C. FINDING MEDICAL LIBRARIES

Overview

In this Appendix, we show you how to quickly find a medical library in your area.

Preparation

Your local public library and medical libraries have interlibrary loan programs with the National Library of Medicine (NLM), one of the largest medical collections in the world. According to the NLM, most of the literature in the general and historical collections of the National Library of Medicine is available on interlibrary loan to any library. If you would like to access NLM medical literature, then visit a library in your area that can request the publications for you.[18]

Finding a Local Medical Library

The quickest method to locate medical libraries is to use the Internet-based directory published by the National Network of Libraries of Medicine (NN/LM). This network includes 4626 members and affiliates that provide many services to librarians, health professionals, and the public. To find a library in your area, simply visit http://nnlm.gov/members/adv.html or call 1-800-338-7657.

Medical Libraries in the U.S. and Canada

In addition to the NN/LM, the National Library of Medicine (NLM) lists a number of libraries with reference facilities that are open to the public. The following is the NLM's list and includes hyperlinks to each library's Web site. These Web pages can provide information on hours of operation and other restrictions. The list below is a small sample of

---

[18] Adapted from the NLM: http://www.nlm.nih.gov/psd/cas/interlibrary.html.

libraries recommended by the National Library of Medicine (sorted alphabetically by name of the U.S. state or Canadian province where the library is located)[19]:

- **Alabama:** Health InfoNet of Jefferson County (Jefferson County Library Cooperative, Lister Hill Library of the Health Sciences), **http://www.uab.edu/infonet/**
- **Alabama:** Richard M. Scrushy Library (American Sports Medicine Institute)
- **Arizona:** Samaritan Regional Medical Center: The Learning Center (Samaritan Health System, Phoenix, Arizona), **http://www.samaritan.edu/library/bannerlibs.htm**
- **California:** Kris Kelly Health Information Center (St. Joseph Health System, Humboldt), **http://www.humboldt1.com/~kkhic/index.html**
- **California:** Community Health Library of Los Gatos, **http://www.healthlib.org/orgresources.html**
- **California:** Consumer Health Program and Services (CHIPS) (County of Los Angeles Public Library, Los Angeles County Harbor-UCLA Medical Center Library) - Carson, CA, **http://www.colapublib.org/services/chips.html**
- **California:** Gateway Health Library (Sutter Gould Medical Foundation)
- **California:** Health Library (Stanford University Medical Center), **http://www-med.stanford.edu/healthlibrary/**
- **California:** Patient Education Resource Center - Health Information and Resources (University of California, San Francisco), **http://sfghdean.ucsf.edu/barnett/PERC/default.asp**
- **California:** Redwood Health Library (Petaluma Health Care District), **http://www.phcd.org/rdwdlib.html**
- **California:** Los Gatos PlaneTree Health Library, **http://planetreesanjose.org/**
- **California:** Sutter Resource Library (Sutter Hospitals Foundation, Sacramento), **http://suttermedicalcenter.org/library/**
- **California:** Health Sciences Libraries (University of California, Davis), **http://www.lib.ucdavis.edu/healthsci/**
- **California:** ValleyCare Health Library & Ryan Comer Cancer Resource Center (ValleyCare Health System, Pleasanton), **http://gaelnet.stmarys-ca.edu/other.libs/gbal/east/vchl.html**
- **California:** Washington Community Health Resource Library (Fremont), **http://www.healthlibrary.org/**
- **Colorado:** William V. Gervasini Memorial Library (Exempla Healthcare), **http://www.saintjosephdenver.org/yourhealth/libraries/**
- **Connecticut:** Hartford Hospital Health Science Libraries (Hartford Hospital), **http://www.harthosp.org/library/**
- **Connecticut:** Healthnet: Connecticut Consumer Health Information Center (University of Connecticut Health Center, Lyman Maynard Stowe Library), **http://library.uchc.edu/departm/hnet/**

---

[19] Abstracted from http://www.nlm.nih.gov/medlineplus/libraries.html.

- **Connecticut:** Waterbury Hospital Health Center Library (Waterbury Hospital, Waterbury), http://www.waterburyhospital.com/library/consumer.shtml
- **Delaware:** Consumer Health Library (Christiana Care Health System, Eugene du Pont Preventive Medicine & Rehabilitation Institute, Wilmington), http://www.christianacare.org/health_guide/health_guide_pmri_health_info.cfm
- **Delaware:** Lewis B. Flinn Library (Delaware Academy of Medicine, Wilmington), http://www.delamed.org/chls.html
- **Georgia:** Family Resource Library (Medical College of Georgia, Augusta), http://cmc.mcg.edu/kids_families/fam_resources/fam_res_lib/frl.htm
- **Georgia:** Health Resource Center (Medical Center of Central Georgia, Macon), http://www.mccg.org/hrc/hrchome.asp
- **Hawaii:** Hawaii Medical Library: Consumer Health Information Service (Hawaii Medical Library, Honolulu), http://hml.org/CHIS/
- **Idaho:** DeArmond Consumer Health Library (Kootenai Medical Center, Coeur d'Alene), http://www.nicon.org/DeArmond/index.htm
- **Illinois:** Health Learning Center of Northwestern Memorial Hospital (Chicago), http://www.nmh.org/health_info/hlc.html
- **Illinois:** Medical Library (OSF Saint Francis Medical Center, Peoria), http://www.osfsaintfrancis.org/general/library/
- **Kentucky:** Medical Library - Services for Patients, Families, Students & the Public (Central Baptist Hospital, Lexington), http://www.centralbap.com/education/community/library.cfm
- **Kentucky:** University of Kentucky - Health Information Library (Chandler Medical Center, Lexington), http://www.mc.uky.edu/PatientEd/
- **Louisiana:** Alton Ochsner Medical Foundation Library (Alton Ochsner Medical Foundation, New Orleans), http://www.ochsner.org/library/
- **Louisiana:** Louisiana State University Health Sciences Center Medical Library-Shreveport, http://lib-sh.lsuhsc.edu/
- **Maine:** Franklin Memorial Hospital Medical Library (Franklin Memorial Hospital, Farmington), http://www.fchn.org/fmh/lib.htm
- **Maine:** Gerrish-True Health Sciences Library (Central Maine Medical Center, Lewiston), http://www.cmmc.org/library/library.html
- **Maine:** Hadley Parrot Health Science Library (Eastern Maine Healthcare, Bangor), http://www.emh.org/hll/hpl/guide.htm
- **Maine:** Maine Medical Center Library (Maine Medical Center, Portland), http://www.mmc.org/library/
- **Maine:** Parkview Hospital (Brunswick), http://www.parkviewhospital.org/
- **Maine:** Southern Maine Medical Center Health Sciences Library (Southern Maine Medical Center, Biddeford), http://www.smmc.org/services/service.php3?choice=10
- **Maine:** Stephens Memorial Hospital's Health Information Library (Western Maine Health, Norway), http://www.wmhcc.org/Library/

- **Manitoba, Canada:** Consumer & Patient Health Information Service (University of Manitoba Libraries), http://www.umanitoba.ca/libraries/units/health/reference/chis.html
- **Manitoba, Canada:** J.W. Crane Memorial Library (Deer Lodge Centre, Winnipeg), http://www.deerlodge.mb.ca/crane_library/about.asp
- **Maryland:** Health Information Center at the Wheaton Regional Library (Montgomery County, Dept. of Public Libraries, Wheaton Regional Library), http://www.mont.lib.md.us/healthinfo/hic.asp
- **Massachusetts:** Baystate Medical Center Library (Baystate Health System), http://www.baystatehealth.com/1024/
- **Massachusetts:** Boston University Medical Center Alumni Medical Library (Boston University Medical Center), http://med-libwww.bu.edu/library/lib.html
- **Massachusetts:** Lowell General Hospital Health Sciences Library (Lowell General Hospital, Lowell), http://www.lowellgeneral.org/library/HomePageLinks/WWW.htm
- **Massachusetts:** Paul E. Woodard Health Sciences Library (New England Baptist Hospital, Boston), http://www.nebh.org/health_lib.asp
- **Massachusetts:** St. Luke's Hospital Health Sciences Library (St. Luke's Hospital, Southcoast Health System, New Bedford), http://www.southcoast.org/library/
- **Massachusetts:** Treadwell Library Consumer Health Reference Center (Massachusetts General Hospital), http://www.mgh.harvard.edu/library/chrcindex.html
- **Massachusetts:** UMass HealthNet (University of Massachusetts Medical School, Worcester), http://healthnet.umassmed.edu/
- **Michigan:** Botsford General Hospital Library - Consumer Health (Botsford General Hospital, Library & Internet Services), http://www.botsfordlibrary.org/consumer.htm
- **Michigan:** Helen DeRoy Medical Library (Providence Hospital and Medical Centers), http://www.providence-hospital.org/library/
- **Michigan:** Marquette General Hospital - Consumer Health Library (Marquette General Hospital, Health Information Center), http://www.mgh.org/center.html
- **Michigan:** Patient Education Resouce Center - University of Michigan Cancer Center (University of Michigan Comprehensive Cancer Center, Ann Arbor), http://www.cancer.med.umich.edu/learn/leares.htm
- **Michigan:** Sladen Library & Center for Health Information Resources - Consumer Health Information (Detroit), http://www.henryford.com/body.cfm?id=39330
- **Montana:** Center for Health Information (St. Patrick Hospital and Health Sciences Center, Missoula)
- **National:** Consumer Health Library Directory (Medical Library Association, Consumer and Patient Health Information Section), http://caphis.mlanet.org/directory/index.html
- **National:** National Network of Libraries of Medicine (National Library of Medicine) - provides library services for health professionals in the United States who do not have access to a medical library, http://nnlm.gov/
- **National:** NN/LM List of Libraries Serving the Public (National Network of Libraries of Medicine), http://nnlm.gov/members/

- **Nevada:** Health Science Library, West Charleston Library (Las Vegas-Clark County Library District, Las Vegas), http://www.lvccld.org/special_collections/medical/index.htm
- **New Hampshire:** Dartmouth Biomedical Libraries (Dartmouth College Library, Hanover), http://www.dartmouth.edu/~biomed/resources.htmld/conshealth.htmld/
- **New Jersey:** Consumer Health Library (Rahway Hospital, Rahway), http://www.rahwayhospital.com/library.htm
- **New Jersey:** Dr. Walter Phillips Health Sciences Library (Englewood Hospital and Medical Center, Englewood), http://www.englewoodhospital.com/links/index.htm
- **New Jersey:** Meland Foundation (Englewood Hospital and Medical Center, Englewood), http://www.geocities.com/ResearchTriangle/9360/
- **New York:** Choices in Health Information (New York Public Library) - NLM Consumer Pilot Project participant, http://www.nypl.org/branch/health/links.html
- **New York:** Health Information Center (Upstate Medical University, State University of New York, Syracuse), http://www.upstate.edu/library/hic/
- **New York:** Health Sciences Library (Long Island Jewish Medical Center, New Hyde Park), http://www.lij.edu/library/library.html
- **New York:** ViaHealth Medical Library (Rochester General Hospital), http://www.nyam.org/library/
- **Ohio:** Consumer Health Library (Akron General Medical Center, Medical & Consumer Health Library), http://www.akrongeneral.org/hwlibrary.htm
- **Oklahoma:** The Health Information Center at Saint Francis Hospital (Saint Francis Health System, Tulsa), http://www.sfh-tulsa.com/services/healthinfo.asp
- **Oregon:** Planetree Health Resource Center (Mid-Columbia Medical Center, The Dalles), http://www.mcmc.net/phrc/
- **Pennsylvania:** Community Health Information Library (Milton S. Hershey Medical Center, Hershey), http://www.hmc.psu.edu/commhealth/
- **Pennsylvania:** Community Health Resource Library (Geisinger Medical Center, Danville), http://www.geisinger.edu/education/commlib.shtml
- **Pennsylvania:** HealthInfo Library (Moses Taylor Hospital, Scranton), http://www.mth.org/healthwellness.html
- **Pennsylvania:** Hopwood Library (University of Pittsburgh, Health Sciences Library System, Pittsburgh), http://www.hsls.pitt.edu/guides/chi/hopwood/index_html
- **Pennsylvania:** Koop Community Health Information Center (College of Physicians of Philadelphia), http://www.collphyphil.org/kooppg1.shtml
- **Pennsylvania:** Learning Resources Center - Medical Library (Susquehanna Health System, Williamsport), http://www.shscares.org/services/lrc/index.asp
- **Pennsylvania:** Medical Library (UPMC Health System, Pittsburgh), http://www.upmc.edu/passavant/library.htm
- **Quebec, Canada:** Medical Library (Montreal General Hospital), http://www.mghlib.mcgill.ca/

- **South Dakota:** Rapid City Regional Hospital Medical Library (Rapid City Regional Hospital), http://www.rcrh.org/Services/Library/Default.asp
- **Texas:** Houston HealthWays (Houston Academy of Medicine-Texas Medical Center Library), http://hhw.library.tmc.edu/
- **Washington:** Community Health Library (Kittitas Valley Community Hospital), http://www.kvch.com/
- **Washington:** Southwest Washington Medical Center Library (Southwest Washington Medical Center, Vancouver), http://www.swmedicalcenter.com/body.cfm?id=72

ONLINE GLOSSARIES

The Internet provides access to a number of free-to-use medical dictionaries. The National Library of Medicine has compiled the following list of online dictionaries:

- ADAM Medical Encyclopedia (A.D.A.M., Inc.), comprehensive medical reference: **http://www.nlm.nih.gov/medlineplus/encyclopedia.html**
- MedicineNet.com Medical Dictionary (MedicineNet, Inc.): **http://www.medterms.com/Script/Main/hp.asp**
- Merriam-Webster Medical Dictionary (Inteli-Health, Inc.): **http://www.intelihealth.com/IH/**
- Multilingual Glossary of Technical and Popular Medical Terms in Eight European Languages (European Commission) - Danish, Dutch, English, French, German, Italian, Portuguese, and Spanish: **http://allserv.rug.ac.be/~rvdstich/eugloss/welcome.html**
- On-line Medical Dictionary (CancerWEB): **http://cancerweb.ncl.ac.uk/omd/**
- Rare Diseases Terms (Office of Rare Diseases): **http://ord.aspensys.com/asp/diseases/diseases.asp**
- Technology Glossary (National Library of Medicine) - Health Care Technology: **http://www.nlm.nih.gov/nichsr/ta101/ta10108.htm**

Beyond these, MEDLINEplus contains a very patient-friendly encyclopedia covering every aspect of medicine (licensed from A.D.A.M., Inc.). The ADAM Medical Encyclopedia can be accessed at **http://www.nlm.nih.gov/medlineplus/encyclopedia.html**. ADAM is also available on commercial Web sites such as drkoop.com (**http://www.drkoop.com/**) and Web MD (**http://my.webmd.com/adam/asset/adam_disease_articles/a_to_z/a**).

Online Dictionary Directories

The following are additional online directories compiled by the National Library of Medicine, including a number of specialized medical dictionaries:

- Medical Dictionaries: Medical & Biological (World Health Organization): **http://www.who.int/hlt/virtuallibrary/English/diction.htm#Medical**
- MEL-Michigan Electronic Library List of Online Health and Medical Dictionaries (Michigan Electronic Library): **http://mel.lib.mi.us/health/health-dictionaries.html**
- Patient Education: Glossaries (DMOZ Open Directory Project): **http://dmoz.org/Health/Education/Patient_Education/Glossaries/**
- Web of Online Dictionaries (Bucknell University): **http://www.yourdictionary.com/diction5.html#medicine**

HYDROXYCITRIC ACID DICTIONARY

The definitions below are derived from official public sources, including the National Institutes of Health [NIH] and the European Union [EU].

Abdominal: Having to do with the abdomen, which is the part of the body between the chest and the hips that contains the pancreas, stomach, intestines, liver, gallbladder, and other organs. [NIH]

Abdominal fat: Fat (adipose tissue) that is centrally distributed between the thorax and pelvis and that induces greater health risk. [NIH]

Acceptor: A substance which, while normally not oxidized by oxygen or reduced by hydrogen, can be oxidized or reduced in presence of a substance which is itself undergoing oxidation or reduction. [NIH]

Adenine: A purine base and a fundamental unit of adenine nucleotides. [NIH]

Adenosine: A nucleoside that is composed of adenine and d-ribose. Adenosine or adenosine derivatives play many important biological roles in addition to being components of DNA and RNA. Adenosine itself is a neurotransmitter. [NIH]

Adenosine Triphosphate: Adenosine 5'-(tetrahydrogen triphosphate). An adenine nucleotide containing three phosphate groups esterified to the sugar moiety. In addition to its crucial roles in metabolism adenosine triphosphate is a neurotransmitter. [NIH]

Adenylate Cyclase: An enzyme of the lyase class that catalyzes the formation of cyclic AMP and pyrophosphate from ATP. EC 4.6.1.1. [NIH]

Adipocytes: Fat-storing cells found mostly in the abdominal cavity and subcutaneous tissue. Fat is usually stored in the form of tryglycerides. [NIH]

Adipose Tissue: Connective tissue composed of fat cells lodged in the meshes of areolar tissue. [NIH]

Afferent: Concerned with the transmission of neural impulse toward the central part of the nervous system. [NIH]

Affinity: 1. Inherent likeness or relationship. 2. A special attraction for a specific element, organ, or structure. 3. Chemical affinity; the force that binds atoms in molecules; the tendency of substances to combine by chemical reaction. 4. The strength of noncovalent chemical binding between two substances as measured by the dissociation constant of the complex. 5. In immunology, a thermodynamic expression of the strength of interaction between a single antigen-binding site and a single antigenic determinant (and thus of the stereochemical compatibility between them), most accurately applied to interactions among simple, uniform antigenic determinants such as haptens. Expressed as the association constant (K litres mole -1), which, owing to the heterogeneity of affinities in a population of antibody molecules of a given specificity, actually represents an average value (mean intrinsic association constant). 6. The reciprocal of the dissociation constant. [EU]

Algorithms: A procedure consisting of a sequence of algebraic formulas and/or logical steps to calculate or determine a given task. [NIH]

Alimentary: Pertaining to food or nutritive material, or to the organs of digestion. [EU]

Alkaline: Having the reactions of an alkali. [EU]

Alternative medicine: Practices not generally recognized by the medical community as standard or conventional medical approaches and used instead of standard treatments.

Alternative medicine includes the taking of dietary supplements, megadose vitamins, and herbal preparations; the drinking of special teas; and practices such as massage therapy, magnet therapy, spiritual healing, and meditation. [NIH]

Aluminum: A metallic element that has the atomic number 13, atomic symbol Al, and atomic weight 26.98. [NIH]

Amino acid: Any organic compound containing an amino (-NH2 and a carboxyl (- COOH) group. The 20 a-amino acids listed in the accompanying table are the amino acids from which proteins are synthesized by formation of peptide bonds during ribosomal translation of messenger RNA; all except glycine, which is not optically active, have the L configuration. Other amino acids occurring in proteins, such as hydroxyproline in collagen, are formed by posttranslational enzymatic modification of amino acids residues in polypeptide chains. There are also several important amino acids, such as the neurotransmitter y-aminobutyric acid, that have no relation to proteins. Abbreviated AA. [EU]

Anions: Negatively charged atoms, radicals or groups of atoms which travel to the anode or positive pole during electrolysis. [NIH]

Anticoagulants: Agents that prevent blood clotting. Naturally occurring agents in the blood are included only when they are used as drugs. [NIH]

Antihypertensive: An agent that reduces high blood pressure. [EU]

Aqueous: Having to do with water. [NIH]

Arteries: The vessels carrying blood away from the heart. [NIH]

Bioavailability: The degree to which a drug or other substance becomes available to the target tissue after administration. [EU]

Bioavailable: The ability of a drug or other substance to be absorbed and used by the body. Orally bioavailable means that a drug or other substance that is taken by mouth can be absorbed and used by the body. [NIH]

Biochemical: Relating to biochemistry; characterized by, produced by, or involving chemical reactions in living organisms. [EU]

Biosynthesis: The building up of a chemical compound in the physiologic processes of a living organism. [EU]

Biotechnology: Body of knowledge related to the use of organisms, cells or cell-derived constituents for the purpose of developing products which are technically, scientifically and clinically useful. Alteration of biologic function at the molecular level (i.e., genetic engineering) is a central focus; laboratory methods used include transfection and cloning technologies, sequence and structure analysis algorithms, computer databases, and gene and protein structure function analysis and prediction. [NIH]

Blood Coagulation: The process of the interaction of blood coagulation factors that results in an insoluble fibrin clot. [NIH]

Blood Platelets: Non-nucleated disk-shaped cells formed in the megakaryocyte and found in the blood of all mammals. They are mainly involved in blood coagulation. [NIH]

Blood pressure: The pressure of blood against the walls of a blood vessel or heart chamber. Unless there is reference to another location, such as the pulmonary artery or one of the heart chambers, it refers to the pressure in the systemic arteries, as measured, for example, in the forearm. [NIH]

Body Fluids: Liquid components of living organisms. [NIH]

Body Mass Index: One of the anthropometric measures of body mass; it has the highest correlation with skinfold thickness or body density. [NIH]

Calcium: A basic element found in nearly all organized tissues. It is a member of the alkaline earth family of metals with the atomic symbol Ca, atomic number 20, and atomic weight 40. Calcium is the most abundant mineral in the body and combines with phosphorus to form calcium phosphate in the bones and teeth. It is essential for the normal functioning of nerves and muscles and plays a role in blood coagulation (as factor IV) and in many enzymatic processes. [NIH]

Carbohydrate: An aldehyde or ketone derivative of a polyhydric alcohol, particularly of the pentahydric and hexahydric alcohols. They are so named because the hydrogen and oxygen are usually in the proportion to form water, $(CH_2O)n$. The most important carbohydrates are the starches, sugars, celluloses, and gums. They are classified into mono-, di-, tri-, poly- and heterosaccharides. [EU]

Carcinogens: Substances that increase the risk of neoplasms in humans or animals. Both genotoxic chemicals, which affect DNA directly, and nongenotoxic chemicals, which induce neoplasms by other mechanism, are included. [NIH]

Cardiovascular: Having to do with the heart and blood vessels. [NIH]

Case report: A detailed report of the diagnosis, treatment, and follow-up of an individual patient. Case reports also contain some demographic information about the patient (for example, age, gender, ethnic origin). [NIH]

Case series: A group or series of case reports involving patients who were given similar treatment. Reports of case series usually contain detailed information about the individual patients. This includes demographic information (for example, age, gender, ethnic origin) and information on diagnosis, treatment, response to treatment, and follow-up after treatment. [NIH]

Cations: Postively charged atoms, radicals or groups of atoms which travel to the cathode or negative pole during electrolysis. [NIH]

Cell: The individual unit that makes up all of the tissues of the body. All living things are made up of one or more cells. [NIH]

Central Nervous System: The main information-processing organs of the nervous system, consisting of the brain, spinal cord, and meninges. [NIH]

Chlorides: Inorganic compounds derived from hydrochloric acid that contain the Cl- ion. [NIH]

Cholesterol: The principal sterol of all higher animals, distributed in body tissues, especially the brain and spinal cord, and in animal fats and oils. [NIH]

Chromium: A trace element that plays a role in glucose metabolism. It has the atomic symbol Cr, atomic number 24, and atomic weight 52. According to the Fourth Annual Report on Carcinogens (NTP85-002,1985), chromium and some of its compounds have been listed as known carcinogens. [NIH]

Citric Acid: A key intermediate in metabolism. It is an acid compound found in citrus fruits. The salts of citric acid (citrates) can be used as anticoagulants due to their calcium chelating ability. [NIH]

Clinical study: A research study in which patients receive treatment in a clinic or other medical facility. Reports of clinical studies can contain results for single patients (case reports) or many patients (case series or clinical trials). [NIH]

Clinical trial: A research study that tests how well new medical treatments or other interventions work in people. Each study is designed to test new methods of screening, prevention, diagnosis, or treatment of a disease. [NIH]

Cloning: The production of a number of genetically identical individuals; in genetic engineering, a process for the efficient replication of a great number of identical DNA molecules. [NIH]

Coenzymes: Substances that are necessary for the action or enhancement of action of an enzyme. Many vitamins are coenzymes. [NIH]

Complement: A term originally used to refer to the heat-labile factor in serum that causes immune cytolysis, the lysis of antibody-coated cells, and now referring to the entire functionally related system comprising at least 20 distinct serum proteins that is the effector not only of immune cytolysis but also of other biologic functions. Complement activation occurs by two different sequences, the classic and alternative pathways. The proteins of the classic pathway are termed 'components of complement' and are designated by the symbols C1 through C9. C1 is a calcium-dependent complex of three distinct proteins C1q, C1r and C1s. The proteins of the alternative pathway (collectively referred to as the properdin system) and complement regulatory proteins are known by semisystematic or trivial names. Fragments resulting from proteolytic cleavage of complement proteins are designated with lower-case letter suffixes, e.g., C3a. Inactivated fragments may be designated with the suffix 'i', e.g. C3bi. Activated components or complexes with biological activity are designated by a bar over the symbol e.g. C1 or C4b,2a. The classic pathway is activated by the binding of C1 to classic pathway activators, primarily antigen-antibody complexes containing IgM, IgG1, IgG3; C1q binds to a single IgM molecule or two adjacent IgG molecules. The alternative pathway can be activated by IgA immune complexes and also by nonimmunologic materials including bacterial endotoxins, microbial polysaccharides, and cell walls. Activation of the classic pathway triggers an enzymatic cascade involving C1, C4, C2 and C3; activation of the alternative pathway triggers a cascade involving C3 and factors B, D and P. Both result in the cleavage of C5 and the formation of the membrane attack complex. Complement activation also results in the formation of many biologically active complement fragments that act as anaphylatoxins, opsonins, or chemotactic factors. [EU]

Complementary and alternative medicine: CAM. Forms of treatment that are used in addition to (complementary) or instead of (alternative) standard treatments. These practices are not considered standard medical approaches. CAM includes dietary supplements, megadose vitamins, herbal preparations, special teas, massage therapy, magnet therapy, spiritual healing, and meditation. [NIH]

Complementary medicine: Practices not generally recognized by the medical community as standard or conventional medical approaches and used to enhance or complement the standard treatments. Complementary medicine includes the taking of dietary supplements, megadose vitamins, and herbal preparations; the drinking of special teas; and practices such as massage therapy, magnet therapy, spiritual healing, and meditation. [NIH]

Computational Biology: A field of biology concerned with the development of techniques for the collection and manipulation of biological data, and the use of such data to make biological discoveries or predictions. This field encompasses all computational methods and theories applicable to molecular biology and areas of computer-based techniques for solving biological problems including manipulation of models and datasets. [NIH]

Contraindications: Any factor or sign that it is unwise to pursue a certain kind of action or treatment, e. g. giving a general anesthetic to a person with pneumonia. [NIH]

Coronary: Encircling in the manner of a crown; a term applied to vessels; nerves, ligaments, etc. The term usually denotes the arteries that supply the heart muscle and, by extension, a pathologic involvement of them. [EU]

Coronary Thrombosis: Presence of a thrombus in a coronary artery, often causing a myocardial infarction. [NIH]

Cortex: The outer layer of an organ or other body structure, as distinguished from the internal substance. [EU]

Curative: Tending to overcome disease and promote recovery. [EU]

Cyclic: Pertaining to or occurring in a cycle or cycles; the term is applied to chemical compounds that contain a ring of atoms in the nucleus. [EU]

Density: The logarithm to the base 10 of the opacity of an exposed and processed film. [NIH]

Deuterium: Deuterium. The stable isotope of hydrogen. It has one neutron and one proton in the nucleus. [NIH]

Developed Countries: Countries that have reached a level of economic achievement through an increase of production, per capita income and consumption, and utilization of natural and human resources. [NIH]

Diagnostic procedure: A method used to identify a disease. [NIH]

Dietary Fiber: The remnants of plant cell walls that are resistant to digestion by the alimentary enzymes of man. It comprises various polysaccharides and lignins. [NIH]

Digestion: The process of breakdown of food for metabolism and use by the body. [NIH]

Dihydroxy: AMPA/Kainate antagonist. [NIH]

Direct: 1. Straight; in a straight line. 2. Performed immediately and without the intervention of subsidiary means. [EU]

Efficacy: The extent to which a specific intervention, procedure, regimen, or service produces a beneficial result under ideal conditions. Ideally, the determination of efficacy is based on the results of a randomized control trial. [NIH]

Electrolyte: A substance that dissociates into ions when fused or in solution, and thus becomes capable of conducting electricity; an ionic solute. [EU]

Electrons: Stable elementary particles having the smallest known negative charge, present in all elements; also called negatrons. Positively charged electrons are called positrons. The numbers, energies and arrangement of electrons around atomic nuclei determine the chemical identities of elements. Beams of electrons are called cathode rays or beta rays, the latter being a high-energy biproduct of nuclear decay. [NIH]

Endotoxic: Of, relating to, or acting as an endotoxin (= a heat-stable toxin, associated with the outer membranes of certain gram-negative bacteria. Endotoxins are not secreted and are released only when the cells are disrupted). [EU]

Energy balance: Energy is the capacity of a body or a physical system for doing work. Energy balance is the state in which the total energy intake equals total energy needs. [NIH]

Enhancer: Transcriptional element in the virus genome. [NIH]

Environmental Health: The science of controlling or modifying those conditions, influences, or forces surrounding man which relate to promoting, establishing, and maintaining health. [NIH]

Enzymatic: Phase where enzyme cuts the precursor protein. [NIH]

Enzyme: A protein that speeds up chemical reactions in the body. [NIH]

Epinephrine: The active sympathomimetic hormone from the adrenal medulla in most species. It stimulates both the alpha- and beta- adrenergic systems, causes systemic vasoconstriction and gastrointestinal relaxation, stimulates the heart, and dilates bronchi and cerebral vessels. It is used in asthma and cardiac failure and to delay absorption of local anesthetics. [NIH]

Ether: One of a class of organic compounds in which any two organic radicals are attached directly to a single oxygen atom. [NIH]

Extracellular: Outside a cell or cells. [EU]

Extraction: The process or act of pulling or drawing out. [EU]

Family Planning: Programs or services designed to assist the family in controlling reproduction by either improving or diminishing fertility. [NIH]

Fat: Total lipids including phospholipids. [NIH]

Fish Products: Food products manufactured from fish (e.g., fish flour, fish meal). [NIH]

Fold: A plication or doubling of various parts of the body. [NIH]

Forskolin: Potent activator of the adenylate cyclase system and the biosynthesis of cyclic AMP. From the plant Coleus forskohlii. Has antihypertensive, positive ionotropic, platelet aggregation inhibitory, and smooth muscle relaxant activities; also lowers intraocular pressure and promotes release of hormones from the pituitary gland. [NIH]

Gallbladder: The pear-shaped organ that sits below the liver. Bile is concentrated and stored in the gallbladder. [NIH]

Gas: Air that comes from normal breakdown of food. The gases are passed out of the body through the rectum (flatus) or the mouth (burp). [NIH]

Gastrointestinal: Refers to the stomach and intestines. [NIH]

Gastrointestinal tract: The stomach and intestines. [NIH]

Gene: The functional and physical unit of heredity passed from parent to offspring. Genes are pieces of DNA, and most genes contain the information for making a specific protein. [NIH]

Gene Expression: The phenotypic manifestation of a gene or genes by the processes of gene action. [NIH]

Glucose: D-Glucose. A primary source of energy for living organisms. It is naturally occurring and is found in fruits and other parts of plants in its free state. It is used therapeutically in fluid and nutrient replacement. [NIH]

Glycogen: A sugar stored in the liver and muscles. It releases glucose into the blood when cells need it for energy. Glycogen is the chief source of stored fuel in the body. [NIH]

Governing Board: The group in which legal authority is vested for the control of health-related institutions and organizations. [NIH]

Hemostasis: The process which spontaneously arrests the flow of blood from vessels carrying blood under pressure. It is accomplished by contraction of the vessels, adhesion and aggregation of formed blood elements, and the process of blood or plasma coagulation. [NIH]

Hepatic: Refers to the liver. [NIH]

Heredity: 1. The genetic transmission of a particular quality or trait from parent to offspring. 2. The genetic constitution of an individual. [EU]

Hormone: A substance in the body that regulates certain organs. Hormones such as gastrin help in breaking down food. Some hormones come from cells in the stomach and small intestine. [NIH]

Hydrochloric Acid: A strong corrosive acid that is commonly used as a laboratory reagent. It is formed by dissolving hydrogen chloride in water. Gastric acid is the hydrochloric acid component of gastric juice. [NIH]

Hydrogen: The first chemical element in the periodic table. It has the atomic symbol H, atomic number 1, and atomic weight 1. It exists, under normal conditions, as a colorless, odorless, tasteless, diatomic gas. Hydrogen ions are protons. Besides the common H1 isotope, hydrogen exists as the stable isotope deuterium and the unstable, radioactive isotope tritium. [NIH]

Hydroxides: Inorganic compounds that contain the OH- group. [NIH]

Hyperlipidemia: An excess of lipids in the blood. [NIH]

Immunogenic: Producing immunity; evoking an immune response. [EU]

In vitro: In the laboratory (outside the body). The opposite of in vivo (in the body). [NIH]

In vivo: In the body. The opposite of in vitro (outside the body or in the laboratory). [NIH]

Infarction: A pathological process consisting of a sudden insufficient blood supply to an area, which results in necrosis of that area. It is usually caused by a thrombus, an embolus, or a vascular torsion. [NIH]

Ingestion: Taking into the body by mouth [NIH]

Insulin: A protein hormone secreted by beta cells of the pancreas. Insulin plays a major role in the regulation of glucose metabolism, generally promoting the cellular utilization of glucose. It is also an important regulator of protein and lipid metabolism. Insulin is used as a drug to control insulin-dependent diabetes mellitus. [NIH]

Insulin-dependent diabetes mellitus: A disease characterized by high levels of blood glucose resulting from defects in insulin secretion, insulin action, or both. Autoimmune, genetic, and environmental factors are involved in the development of type I diabetes. [NIH]

Intestines: The section of the alimentary canal from the stomach to the anus. It includes the large intestine and small intestine. [NIH]

Intracellular: Inside a cell. [NIH]

Intraocular: Within the eye. [EU]

Intraocular pressure: Pressure of the fluid inside the eye; normal IOP varies among individuals. [NIH]

Ions: An atom or group of atoms that have a positive or negative electric charge due to a gain (negative charge) or loss (positive charge) of one or more electrons. Atoms with a positive charge are known as cations; those with a negative charge are anions. [NIH]

Islet: Cell producing insulin in pancreas. [NIH]

Kb: A measure of the length of DNA fragments, 1 Kb = 1000 base pairs. The largest DNA fragments are up to 50 kilobases long. [NIH]

Leptin: A 16-kD peptide hormone secreted from white adipocytes and implicated in the regulation of food intake and energy balance. Leptin provides the key afferent signal from fat cells in the feedback system that controls body fat stores. [NIH]

Lipid: Fat. [NIH]

Lipid A: Lipid A is the biologically active component of lipopolysaccharides. It shows strong endotoxic activity and exhibits immunogenic properties. [NIH]

Lipopolysaccharides: Substance consisting of polysaccharide and lipid. [NIH]

Liver: A large, glandular organ located in the upper abdomen. The liver cleanses the blood and aids in digestion by secreting bile. [NIH]

Meat: The edible portions of any animal used for food including domestic mammals (the major ones being cattle, swine, and sheep) along with poultry, fish, shellfish, and game. [NIH]

Mediator: An object or substance by which something is mediated, such as (1) a structure of the nervous system that transmits impulses eliciting a specific response; (2) a chemical substance (transmitter substance) that induces activity in an excitable tissue, such as nerve or muscle; or (3) a substance released from cells as the result of the interaction of antigen with antibody or by the action of antigen with a sensitized lymphocyte. [EU]

MEDLINE: An online database of MEDLARS, the computerized bibliographic Medical Literature Analysis and Retrieval System of the National Library of Medicine. [NIH]

Melanin: The substance that gives the skin its color. [NIH]

Membranes: Thin layers of tissue which cover parts of the body, separate adjacent cavities, or connect adjacent structures. [NIH]

Methanol: A colorless, flammable liquid used in the manufacture of formaldehyde and acetic acid, in chemical synthesis, antifreeze, and as a solvent. Ingestion of methanol is toxic and may cause blindness. [NIH]

MI: Myocardial infarction. Gross necrosis of the myocardium as a result of interruption of the blood supply to the area; it is almost always caused by atherosclerosis of the coronary arteries, upon which coronary thrombosis is usually superimposed. [NIH]

Micronutrients: Essential dietary elements or organic compounds that are required in only small quantities for normal physiologic processes to occur. [NIH]

Microorganism: An organism that can be seen only through a microscope. Microorganisms include bacteria, protozoa, algae, and fungi. Although viruses are not considered living organisms, they are sometimes classified as microorganisms. [NIH]

Molecular: Of, pertaining to, or composed of molecules : a very small mass of matter. [EU]

Molecule: A chemical made up of two or more atoms. The atoms in a molecule can be the same (an oxygen molecule has two oxygen atoms) or different (a water molecule has two hydrogen atoms and one oxygen atom). Biological molecules, such as proteins and DNA, can be made up of many thousands of atoms. [NIH]

Motility: The ability to move spontaneously. [EU]

Myocardium: The muscle tissue of the heart composed of striated, involuntary muscle known as cardiac muscle. [NIH]

Necrosis: A pathological process caused by the progressive degradative action of enzymes that is generally associated with severe cellular trauma. It is characterized by mitochondrial swelling, nuclear flocculation, uncontrolled cell lysis, and ultimately cell death. [NIH]

Neurotransmitter: Any of a group of substances that are released on excitation from the axon terminal of a presynaptic neuron of the central or peripheral nervous system and travel across the synaptic cleft to either excite or inhibit the target cell. Among the many substances that have the properties of a neurotransmitter are acetylcholine, norepinephrine, epinephrine, dopamine, glycine, y-aminobutyrate, glutamic acid, substance P, enkephalins, endorphins, and serotonin. [EU]

Niacin: Water-soluble vitamin of the B complex occurring in various animal and plant tissues. Required by the body for the formation of coenzymes NAD and NADP. Has pellagra-curative, vasodilating, and antilipemic properties. [NIH]

Overweight: An excess of body weight but not necessarily body fat; a body mass index of 25 to 29.9 kg/m2. [NIH]

Oxidation: The act of oxidizing or state of being oxidized. Chemically it consists in the increase of positive charges on an atom or the loss of negative charges. Most biological oxidations are accomplished by the removal of a pair of hydrogen atoms (dehydrogenation) from a molecule. Such oxidations must be accompanied by reduction of an acceptor molecule. Univalent o. indicates loss of one electron; divalent o., the loss of two electrons. [EU]

Pancreas: A mixed exocrine and endocrine gland situated transversely across the posterior abdominal wall in the epigastric and hypochondriac regions. The endocrine portion is comprised of the Islets of Langerhans, while the exocrine portion is a compound acinar gland that secretes digestive enzymes. [NIH]

Pelvis: The lower part of the abdomen, located between the hip bones. [NIH]

Peptide: Any compound consisting of two or more amino acids, the building blocks of proteins. Peptides are combined to make proteins. [NIH]

Pharmacologic: Pertaining to pharmacology or to the properties and reactions of drugs. [EU]

Phenylalanine: An aromatic amino acid that is essential in the animal diet. It is a precursor of melanin, dopamine, noradrenalin, and thyroxine. [NIH]

Phospholipids: Lipids containing one or more phosphate groups, particularly those derived from either glycerol (phosphoglycerides; glycerophospholipids) or sphingosine (sphingolipids). They are polar lipids that are of great importance for the structure and function of cell membranes and are the most abundant of membrane lipids, although not stored in large amounts in the system. [NIH]

Phosphorus: A non-metallic element that is found in the blood, muscles, nevers, bones, and teeth, and is a component of adenosine triphosphate (ATP; the primary energy source for the body's cells.) [NIH]

Physiologic: Having to do with the functions of the body. When used in the phrase "physiologic age," it refers to an age assigned by general health, as opposed to calendar age. [NIH]

Pituitary Gland: A small, unpaired gland situated in the sella turcica tissue. It is connected to the hypothalamus by a short stalk. [NIH]

Plasma: The clear, yellowish, fluid part of the blood that carries the blood cells. The proteins that form blood clots are in plasma. [NIH]

Platelet Aggregation: The attachment of platelets to one another. This clumping together can be induced by a number of agents (e.g., thrombin, collagen) and is part of the mechanism leading to the formation of a thrombus. [NIH]

Pneumonia: Inflammation of the lungs. [NIH]

Potassium: An element that is in the alkali group of metals. It has an atomic symbol K, atomic number 19, and atomic weight 39.10. It is the chief cation in the intracellular fluid of muscle and other cells. Potassium ion is a strong electrolyte and it plays a significant role in the regulation of fluid volume and maintenance of the water-electrolyte balance. [NIH]

Practice Guidelines: Directions or principles presenting current or future rules of policy for the health care practitioner to assist him in patient care decisions regarding diagnosis, therapy, or related clinical circumstances. The guidelines may be developed by government agencies at any level, institutions, professional societies, governing boards, or by the convening of expert panels. The guidelines form a basis for the evaluation of all aspects of health care and delivery. [NIH]

Precursor: Something that precedes. In biological processes, a substance from which another, usually more active or mature substance is formed. In clinical medicine, a sign or symptom that heralds another. [EU]

Protein S: The vitamin K-dependent cofactor of activated protein C. Together with protein C, it inhibits the action of factors VIIIa and Va. A deficiency in protein S can lead to recurrent venous and arterial thrombosis. [NIH]

Proteins: Polymers of amino acids linked by peptide bonds. The specific sequence of amino acids determines the shape and function of the protein. [NIH]

Protons: Stable elementary particles having the smallest known positive charge, found in the nuclei of all elements. The proton mass is less than that of a neutron. A proton is the nucleus of the light hydrogen atom, i.e., the hydrogen ion. [NIH]

Public Policy: A course or method of action selected, usually by a government, from among alternatives to guide and determine present and future decisions. [NIH]

Radioactive: Giving off radiation. [NIH]

Randomized: Describes an experiment or clinical trial in which animal or human subjects are assigned by chance to separate groups that compare different treatments. [NIH]

Receptor: A molecule inside or on the surface of a cell that binds to a specific substance and causes a specific physiologic effect in the cell. [NIH]

Receptors, Serotonin: Cell-surface proteins that bind serotonin and trigger intracellular changes which influence the behavior of cells. Several types of serotonin receptors have been recognized which differ in their pharmacology, molecular biology, and mode of action. [NIH]

Refer: To send or direct for treatment, aid, information, de decision. [NIH]

Regimen: A treatment plan that specifies the dosage, the schedule, and the duration of treatment. [NIH]

Relaxant: 1. Lessening or reducing tension. 2. An agent that lessens tension. [EU]

Ribose: A pentose active in biological systems usually in its D-form. [NIH]

Screening: Checking for disease when there are no symptoms. [NIH]

Seafood: Marine fish and shellfish used as food or suitable for food. (Webster, 3d ed) shellfish and fish products are more specific types of seafood. [NIH]

Sedentary: 1. Sitting habitually; of inactive habits. 2. Pertaining to a sitting posture. [EU]

Serotonin: A biochemical messenger and regulator, synthesized from the essential amino acid L-tryptophan. In humans it is found primarily in the central nervous system, gastrointestinal tract, and blood platelets. Serotonin mediates several important physiological functions including neurotransmission, gastrointestinal motility, hemostasis, and cardiovascular integrity. Multiple receptor families (receptors, serotonin) explain the broad physiological actions and distribution of this biochemical mediator. [NIH]

Serum: The clear liquid part of the blood that remains after blood cells and clotting proteins have been removed. [NIH]

Smooth muscle: Muscle that performs automatic tasks, such as constricting blood vessels. [NIH]

Sodium: An element that is a member of the alkali group of metals. It has the atomic symbol Na, atomic number 11, and atomic weight 23. With a valence of 1, it has a strong affinity for oxygen and other nonmetallic elements. Sodium provides the chief cation of the extracellular body fluids. Its salts are the most widely used in medicine. (From Dorland, 27th ed) Physiologically the sodium ion plays a major role in blood pressure regulation, maintenance of fluid volume, and electrolyte balance. [NIH]

Solvent: 1. Dissolving; effecting a solution. 2. A liquid that dissolves or that is capable of dissolving; the component of a solution that is present in greater amount. [EU]

Specialist: In medicine, one who concentrates on 1 special branch of medical science. [NIH]

Species: A taxonomic category subordinate to a genus (or subgenus) and superior to a subspecies or variety, composed of individuals possessing common characters distinguishing them from other categories of individuals of the same taxonomic level. In taxonomic nomenclature, species are designated by the genus name followed by a Latin or Latinized adjective or noun. [EU]

Spinal cord: The main trunk or bundle of nerves running down the spine through holes in the spinal bone (the vertebrae) from the brain to the level of the lower back. [NIH]

Stomach: An organ of digestion situated in the left upper quadrant of the abdomen between the termination of the esophagus and the beginning of the duodenum. [NIH]

Subspecies: A category intermediate in rank between species and variety, based on a smaller number of correlated characters than are used to differentiate species and generally conditioned by geographical and/or ecological occurrence. [NIH]

Substrate: A substance upon which an enzyme acts. [EU]

Suppression: A conscious exclusion of disapproved desire contrary with repression, in which the process of exclusion is not conscious. [NIH]

Synergistic: Acting together; enhancing the effect of another force or agent. [EU]

Thorax: A part of the trunk between the neck and the abdomen; the chest. [NIH]

Thyroid: A gland located near the windpipe (trachea) that produces thyroid hormone, which helps regulate growth and metabolism. [NIH]

Tissue: A group or layer of cells that are alike in type and work together to perform a specific function. [NIH]

Toxic: Having to do with poison or something harmful to the body. Toxic substances usually cause unwanted side effects. [NIH]

Toxicology: The science concerned with the detection, chemical composition, and pharmacologic action of toxic substances or poisons and the treatment and prevention of toxic manifestations. [NIH]

Trace element: Substance or element essential to plant or animal life, but present in extremely small amounts. [NIH]

Transfection: The uptake of naked or purified DNA into cells, usually eukaryotic. It is analogous to bacterial transformation. [NIH]

Translocation: The movement of material in solution inside the body of the plant. [NIH]

Tryptophan: An essential amino acid that is necessary for normal growth in infants and for nitrogen balance in adults. It is a precursor serotonin and niacin. [NIH]

Tyrosine: A non-essential amino acid. In animals it is synthesized from phenylalanine. It is also the precursor of epinephrine, thyroid hormones, and melanin. [NIH]

Urbanization: The process whereby a society changes from a rural to an urban way of life. It refers also to the gradual increase in the proportion of people living in urban areas. [NIH]

Veterinary Medicine: The medical science concerned with the prevention, diagnosis, and treatment of diseases in animals. [NIH]

Virus: Submicroscopic organism that causes infectious disease. In cancer therapy, some viruses may be made into vaccines that help the body build an immune response to, and kill, tumor cells. [NIH]

Vitro: Descriptive of an event or enzyme reaction under experimental investigation occurring outside a living organism. Parts of an organism or microorganism are used together with artificial substrates and/or conditions. [NIH]

Vivo: Outside of or removed from the body of a living organism. [NIH]

INDEX

A
Abdominal, 10, 43, 51
Abdominal fat, 10, 43
Acceptor, 43, 50
Adenine, 43
Adenosine, 20, 43, 51
Adenosine Triphosphate, 20, 43, 51
Adenylate Cyclase, 43, 48
Adipocytes, 43, 49
Adipose Tissue, 43
Afferent, 43, 49
Affinity, 43, 52
Algorithms, 43, 44
Alimentary, 43, 47, 49
Alkaline, 43, 45
Alternative medicine, 43
Aluminum, 11, 44
Amino acid, 44, 51, 52, 53
Anions, 44, 49
Anticoagulants, 44, 45
Antihypertensive, 44, 48
Aqueous, 17, 21, 44
Arteries, 44, 46, 50

B
Bioavailability, 20, 44
Bioavailable, 19, 20, 44
Biochemical, 44, 52
Biosynthesis, 44, 48
Biotechnology, 3, 27, 44
Blood Coagulation, 44, 45
Blood Platelets, 44, 52
Blood pressure, 44, 52
Body Fluids, 44, 52
Body Mass Index, 19, 20, 44, 50

C
Calcium, 4, 18, 21, 45, 46
Carbohydrate, 10, 18, 45
Carcinogens, 45
Cardiovascular, 45, 52
Case report, 45
Case series, 45
Cations, 45, 49
Cell, 6, 20, 44, 45, 46, 47, 48, 49, 50, 51, 52
Central Nervous System, 45, 52
Chlorides, 17, 45
Cholesterol, 17, 18, 20, 45
Chromium, 10, 20, 45
Citric Acid, 16, 45

Clinical study, 20, 45
Clinical trial, 3, 27, 45, 52
Cloning, 44, 45
Coenzymes, 46, 50
Complement, 46
Complementary and alternative medicine, 9, 13, 46
Complementary medicine, 9, 46
Computational Biology, 27, 46
Contraindications, ii, 46
Coronary, 46, 50
Coronary Thrombosis, 46, 50
Cortex, 6, 10, 46
Curative, 47, 50
Cyclic, 43, 47, 48

D
Density, 44, 47
Deuterium, 47, 49
Developed Countries, 20, 47
Diagnostic procedure, 15, 47
Dietary Fiber, 19, 47
Digestion, 43, 47, 49, 53
Dihydroxy, 16, 47
Direct, iii, 47, 52

E
Efficacy, 20, 47
Electrolyte, 47, 51, 52
Electrons, 47, 49, 50
Endotoxic, 47, 49
Energy balance, 47, 49
Enhancer, 18, 47
Environmental Health, 26, 28, 47
Enzymatic, 44, 45, 46, 47
Enzyme, 18, 20, 43, 46, 47, 53
Epinephrine, 47, 50, 53
Ether, 16, 47
Extracellular, 20, 48, 52
Extraction, 17, 48

F
Family Planning, 27, 48
Fat, 4, 10, 17, 18, 19, 20, 43, 48, 49, 50
Fish Products, 48, 52
Fold, 20, 48
Forskolin, 19, 48

G
Gallbladder, 43, 48
Gas, 48
Gastrointestinal, 20, 47, 48, 52

Gastrointestinal tract, 48, 52
Gene, 10, 44, 48
Gene Expression, 10, 48
Glucose, 45, 48, 49
Glycogen, 18, 48
Governing Board, 48, 51
H
Hemostasis, 48, 52
Hepatic, 20, 48
Heredity, 48
Hormone, 47, 48, 49, 53
Hydrochloric Acid, 45, 48
Hydrogen, 16, 43, 45, 47, 48, 50, 52
Hydroxides, 17, 49
Hyperlipidemia, 18, 49
I
Immunogenic, 49
In vitro, 11, 20, 49
In vivo, 11, 49
Infarction, 46, 49, 50
Ingestion, 4, 11, 49, 50
Insulin, 10, 49
Insulin-dependent diabetes mellitus, 49
Intestines, 43, 48, 49
Intracellular, 20, 49, 51, 52
Intraocular, 48, 49
Intraocular pressure, 48, 49
Ions, 17, 47, 48, 49
Islet, 11, 49
K
Kb, 26, 49
L
Leptin, 10, 20, 49
Lipid, 10, 17, 18, 49
Lipid A, 17, 49
Lipopolysaccharides, 49
Liver, 43, 48, 49
M
Meat, 18, 49
Mediator, 49, 52
MEDLINE, 27, 50
Melanin, 50, 51, 53
Membranes, 20, 47, 50, 51
Methanol, 16, 50
MI, 41, 50
Micronutrients, 20, 50
Microorganism, 50, 53
Molecular, 10, 11, 27, 29, 44, 46, 50, 52
Molecule, 16, 46, 50, 52
Motility, 50, 52
Myocardium, 50

N
Necrosis, 49, 50
Neurotransmitter, 43, 44, 50
Niacin, 10, 50, 53
O
Overweight, 6, 18, 21, 50
Oxidation, 9, 10, 20, 43, 50
P
Pancreas, 43, 49, 51
Pelvis, 43, 51
Peptide, 44, 49, 51
Pharmacologic, 51, 53
Phenylalanine, 51, 53
Phospholipids, 48, 51
Phosphorus, 45, 51
Physiologic, 44, 50, 51, 52
Pituitary Gland, 48, 51
Plasma, 18, 48, 51
Platelet Aggregation, 48, 51
Pneumonia, 46, 51
Potassium, 4, 18, 20, 21, 51
Practice Guidelines, 28, 51
Precursor, 47, 51, 53
Protein S, 44, 51
Proteins, 44, 46, 50, 51, 52
Protons, 48, 52
Public Policy, 27, 52
R
Radioactive, 49, 52
Randomized, 11, 47, 52
Receptor, 52
Receptors, Serotonin, 52
Refer, 1, 46, 52
Regimen, 47, 52
Relaxant, 48, 52
Ribose, 43, 52
S
Screening, 45, 52
Seafood, 18, 52
Sedentary, 21, 52
Serotonin, 6, 10, 20, 50, 52, 53
Serum, 10, 18, 20, 46, 52
Smooth muscle, 48, 52
Sodium, 18, 52
Solvent, 17, 50, 52
Specialist, 33, 52
Species, 17, 18, 47, 52, 53
Spinal cord, 45, 53
Stomach, 43, 48, 49, 53
Subspecies, 52, 53
Substrate, 9, 53
Suppression, 6, 11, 53

Synergistic, 18, 53
T
Thorax, 43, 53
Thyroid, 53
Tissue, 43, 44, 50, 51, 53
Toxic, iv, 50, 53
Toxicology, 4, 28, 53
Trace element, 45, 53
Transfection, 44, 53
Translocation, 11, 53

Tryptophan, 52, 53
Tyrosine, 18, 53
U
Urbanization, 21, 53
V
Veterinary Medicine, 27, 53
Virus, 47, 53
Vitro, 53
Vivo, 53